I WON'T BE CRIPPLED WHEN I SEE JESUS

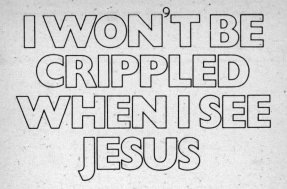

I WON'T BE CRIPPLED WHEN I SEE JESUS

EVERETT PAYTON

KINGSWAY PUBLICATIONS
EASTBOURNE

ISBN 0 86065 119 3

Printed in Great Britain for
KINGSWAY PUBLICATIONS LTD
Lottbridge Drove, Eastbourne, E. Sussex BN23 6NT by
Richard Clay (The Chaucer Press) Ltd, Bungay, Suffolk

This book is dedicated to my wife Mary Lee,
who has been an inspiration to the Payton family.
She reflects the image of the untiring and beloved
woman described in Proverbs 31.

Together we dedicate this book to the glory of God,
who told us this story through Everett Lee.

Contents

Introduction

"Not one of us lives for himself, and not one dies for himself" (Rom. 14:7). You and I are unique individuals, and our lives touch many other lives. More profoundly than we may know, each of us has an impact on others.

This is the story of a young boy named Everett Lee, an uncommon child born into a common family. A thick jungle of water-on-the-brain, blindness, and cerebral palsy surrounded his crib. Yet God knew the way through the Payton family's wilderness of hurt, fear, and uncertainty.

The life of a handicapped boy makes lasting impressions on the people around him. Those people, likewise, have a strong effect on the life of a crippled boy. Often the marks are painful and permanent. Our son taught us that God intends to make etchings of lasting beauty through the gift of a special child.

In the eventful span of nine years, the living God by invitation added new dimensions to our lives. Everett Lee was the agent by which we grew. Our faith was expanded by this baby with the misshaped head. His blind eyes came to have inspiring spiritual vision. "Normal" children and adults were constantly challenged by the uncrippled spirit of this smiling boy with feeble legs. He deeply touched many lives. When God took Everett Lee from our home to his, he perfected all of our son's imperfections.

The message of Everett Lee's life is a happy one. It reveals the power of God to bring victory from despair. An accomplished writer could have told this story better. An observer from outside his family would have much to say. However, I want you to witness this story from a front-row seat.

My name is Everett, also. I am "Daddy" to this young man, whom the heavenly Father used to lead me. Everett Lee reached out with a withered hand to the dad who often was more "crippled" than he. Although a Christian minister, I regularly "saw" less than my blind boy. But he was patient, and the Lord was, too.

The family in the parsonage knows the same anxiety and agony as does your family. We are susceptible to the same infections of attitude and spirit. So please read these chapters with assurance that real fears and real joys are being shared. These are the genuine feelings in which God can work.

Everett means "strong and brave." God entered into this boy's weakness and showed himself strong. He gave our son courage out of confidence and hope in Jesus Christ. The Everett who is writing this story does so in dependence on that same faithful source.

Special thanks go to Mrs. Shirley Harpool and Mrs. Judy Parmley, who have aided substantially in this effort. I also am grateful to Liberty Christian Church for allowing me time away from the pastorate to prepare this record. Each of these and our family pray that you may be encouraged and instructed by the life of Everett Lee Payton, God's perfect gift to us. God knows the way through your wilderness, too!

EVERETT J. PAYTON

CHAPTER ONE

Crisis

WHAT DO YOU DO when the speedometer registers 90 miles per hour and you come upon a radar speed trap?

"Father, you know all about Everett Lee. Please don't let the police delay us."

How I wished the little man in his mother's lap would make some bright, childish quip. He always came up with something, sometimes funny and sometimes embarrassing, especially if his daddy did something wrong. But he was in no condition to do that now.

I kept the needle pegged, my foot firmly on the accelerator. As we shot past two state patrolmen, their heads snapped around. We descended the north side of Rex Hill, continuing toward Portland.

Our trip had begun at 6:15 A.M., just as the first rays of sunlight were breaking through the gray fall mist in the Willamette Valley. Our son Fred had just come in from his paper route, which covered the entire town of Yamhill, Oregon. When he'd entered the bedroom, he'd discovered his brother in the middle of a seizure.

Seizures were a new development in the life of a very special boy. Everett Lee had been born with a condition termed "hydrocephalus." This strange word simply indicates a buildup of pressure caused by excess fluid in the head. His hydrocephalus had caused blindness and cerebral palsy. We learned these terms and others while facing life together with him.

Now excessive pressure in his head was triggering seizures. Once before the built-up pressure had turned off the entire nervous system of this four-year-old. Seizures were a meter of what was happening inside his head, signaling that he was in trouble.

Fred sounded the alarm throughout the house, and Everett Lee was quickly gathered into his mother's arms. I rushed to dress and start the car. We shared a brief but fervent prayer. "Father, please protect Everett Lee and us as we drive."

As we got into the car, we saw the brave and tear-stained faces of Kathy, Jo Ann, and Fred watching from the window. The girls were now seven and nine years old. Their big brother was twelve. Already these young ones, along with their mother Mary Lee and me, had learned from similar crucial moments that the bundled boy in Mother's lap was a gift from God that bound us together in a special trust of love and prayer.

We threw gravel from the driveway, starting up Main Street toward Portland, 40 miles to the north. Soon we flashed by the house on the opposite side of town where the Eckrode family was already preparing to care for our children. How thankful we were for this understanding family. They had an extra capacity to understand, because God had trusted them with a special child who, like Everett Lee, was blind and palsied.

I drove as fast as possible through the beautiful hilly countryside. Eleven miles toward our destination, we reached Newberg, a sedate community of 5000. There was hardly another car on the streets, but we broke the early morning tranquility as we sped through.

Suddenly I decided to stop at the little hospital there. Everett Lee looked bad to me. Mary Lee had placed her fingers between his teeth to protect him and to assist his breathing, and he had nearly bitten them through. Good Samaritan Hospital in Portland was the only place in northern Oregon equipped to meet Everett Lee's needs fully, but we were desperate to receive some temporary help. A quick U-turn took us down a side street and into the empty hospital parking lot.

I dashed into the emergency room. No one was in sight. I shouted, "Is there anyone home?" My mind was racing; seconds seemed like an eternity. When I received no immediate response, I decided we should drive on to Portland without further delay. Everett Lee was in serious trouble.

A city police car was waiting beside ours as I came out of the hospital. The policeman had seen us speed into the hospital lot. When he recognized our circumstances, he put the "coupon book" aside, but refused to provide an escort.

So we were back on the road, hurtling toward our rendezvous with the radar patrolmen. Mary Lee, her aching fingers yet clenched in Everett Lee's jaw, was in prayer for him and for me as I drove. I prayed for the two of them. They were both suffering. Seeing my concern, Mary Lee assured me, "God has always been good to us. He will see us through now, as well."

When I see the quiet beauty of a mother holding her baby, I often think of Madonna and Child paintings in which the travail of birth is lost in the peaceful strength of motherhood. I looked upon my Mary now. Enduring pain nearly as intense as that of childbirth, she had a Madonna-like quality.

Five miles beyond the radar unit, a state patrolman with red lights flashing and siren blaring pulled us over. I ran back to him, described our emergency, and requested an escort. He looked into the car and saw that my tale was true.

"Go ahead," he said. "Two cars traveling at high speed are more dangerous than one traveling alone. Be careful." He wished us well, and I tromped the accelerator again. It is likely that he radioed ahead of our plight, because we weren't stopped again.

As we neared the hospital, we prayed, "Father,

thank you for the dedicated ministry of the medical profession which you have supplied in Everett Lee's times of need."

Through Everett Lee's life we had grown to know the exciting power and goodness of our God. We pointed constantly to him as the source of the peace and blessing we had experienced. In our praise to him, we included thanks for his servants in the medical profession.

On this occasion Everett Lee responded well to the tender care supplied by God through physicians and nurses. Surgery relieved the pressure on Everett Lee's brain, and in a few days he came home to bless our family and to touch many lives with an extra measure of God's grace.

It seems incredible to us as we savor how much God stretched our lives through this young boy. Through tears and laughter, our faith and love grew. In this boy God illustrated much of what he intends us all to know. "Father, thank you again for Everett Lee, a perfect gift in imperfect wrapping."

Come with me back to the time when his life began.

CHAPTER TWO

Festive Birth

THE ROSE FESTIVAL is the big event of the year in Portland. It is a little like the Mardi Gras in New Orleans, the Chinese New Year in San Francisco, or the St. Patrick's Day festivities in Chicago. It is more like the Pasadena Tournament of Roses, with a similarly beautiful rose parade. Months of preparation precede the 10 days of activities in June.

This June we were planning our own festivities. The Paytons were in full preparation to receive a new baby to complete our family. Our physician was in Portland, and Mary Lee's mother had served as an R.N. in the nursery department of a Portland hospital for more than 20 years. We were pleased that the city had generously planned a celebration to commemorate our big event.

When Kathy had been born, we'd been alarmed

at snow and flood conditions that forced many road closures. Everett Lee's choice, though, was much better. We had no fear of road closures or weather hazards in June.

It was only a short drive to Portland from Woodburn, the fast-growing community that had become our home three years earlier. We had driven that stretch of freeway often, because both sets of our parents and Mary Lee's two sisters and their families lived in Portland.

Mary Lee's health had been very good throughout this pregnancy. Our church was thriving. We had just occupied a fine new church building. God was already framing our lives in his goodness and supplying spiritual strength for the days ahead.

We had selected the child's name (providing he cooperated by being a boy) by combining our two names. This choice seemed then to be rather coincidental, but later we would see that God was guiding our selection. This name would come to inspire Everett Lee and have great meaning for those who knew him.

We began to receive indicators that our fourth child was on his way. The doctor recommended that we come to his office to verify the progress toward birth. Mary Lee had been through this process three times. To her amazement, the symptoms were diagnosed as false labor. Perplexed, we returned to her parents' house, where she spent a fitful night. Her severe pain was somehow different from her usual preliminary labor pains. We assumed all of this must indeed be false labor.

June 10 was a beautiful Saturday morning for the Grand Floral Parade. The whole family was in town. We decided to join the throngs and witness the pageantry on the streets. Mary Lee was still hurting, but she was a trooper. If this gnawing pain was false labor, it was not going to prevent her from enjoying the parade with her family.

Enjoy it we did, laughing at the thought of how many among the half a million spectators were having labor pains. Our kids were thrilled at the bands, the lovely floats, and the horses. They were not aware of how tightly Mommy squeezed Daddy's hand intermittently in those hours. As the day wore on, we knew it would end with the delivery of our child. Anticipation made the excitement of the day's spectacle even greater.

Following another call to the doctor, we bade our youngsters good-bye at their grandparents' house. At last the wonder of the partnership with God in giving a new life was about to be completed. Mary Lee was clearly showing fatigue from the day's activity plus 24 hours of pain.

Had we known what we learned that night, Mary Lee probably would have refrained from sharing in the public extravaganza. She was not in false labor. The labor was not progressing as usual, but she was in actual labor all of that time. We would not understand until the next day what was causing this birth to be different.

As we crossed the city on the 20-minute drive to the warm hospitality of Good Samaritan, pictures of the crowds and bands were still flashing in our minds. Almost too quickly we arrived at the hospital for the unequal sharing of husband and wife in childbirth.

Saturday night slipped away and, in our attentiveness to God and each other, Sunday began almost unnoticed. I knew something was wrong. Mary Lee was hurting too much and not making progress.

Out of frustration and fear, I called the doctor into conference. Ministers are supposed to have a respectful deference to doctors, especially on their home turf in the hospital. But my professionalism wore thin in the wee hours of that morning.

I knew the person in that bed very well, and I loved her deeply. The hand I held belonged to a wonderfully strong and brave woman with a trust in God that always had been a challenge to my own. And I knew she was in trouble.

As morning approached, my prayers took a startling new direction. "Father, please don't let her die. We all love and need her too much. Please don't let her die."

The doctor knew Mary Lee's courage, too. He had been her family physician as far back as grade school, when he nursed her through rheumatic fever. As he saw her condition eroding further, he acknowledged the presence of a factor which he did not understand. A specialist was called. After a careful examination, the specialist directed that Mary Lee be immediately prepared for a cesarean section. It was almost morning. Her condition was grave.

Almost morning! Sunday morning! I should let the church know what was happening. The people would want to pray for our needs, and they would have to make some provision for the worship services. So while Mary Lee was being prepared for surgery, I placed the call to Alton Douthit, chairman of the elders.

He was very comforting to me. What a ministry one person can have in a brief moment when the Spirit of God expresses himself through that individual. Alton said he would cover for me in the pulpit and promised the congregation's prayers for us. Many later reported to me that God gave Alton a wonderful message that day. On this morning God blessed Alton mightily and made him a great blessing as well.

Throughout my long wait, a verse occurred and recurred to me. Midway in Psalm 30 the Lord says, "Weeping may last for a night, but a shout of joy comes in the morning." I claimed that promise of our Lord.

At last Everett Lee was born. It was nearly 8:00 A.M.

Waves of joy swept over me. God had fulfilled his promise. Joy had come in the morning light of God's faithfulness.

That morning became a major turning point for me. I began personalizing the Word of God in my life. The claiming of God's precious promises became for our family and for Everett Lee himself the greatest source of God's strength in our lives.

Throughout the period of extended labor, I understood how much my wife meant to me. My love for my children's mother had grown even as her strength had waned. The doctor said the baby's large head had made normal birth impossible from the beginning, but I hardly heard him. I could only cry out in the most sincere gratitude I have ever known, "Father, thank you for protecting my Mary Lee, and thank you for our new son."

CHAPTER THREE

Hydro What?

"**H**YDROCEPHALUS! Doctor, what is that?"

"It is a condition of excess spinal fluid in the head, which causes the head to be enlarged."

My thoughts ran wild at this news. Images of tragic little children pictured in the "horror" pages of textbooks were flashing before me. I recalled their being described as "water-head babies," hopeless little beings sent to institutions to live out a vegetable-like existence.

Questions came tumbling out. "Doctor, what does this mean? What caused this? Will our baby live? Will he be all right?"

The doctor to whom I was speaking was a highly specialized neurosurgeon. That night we had gone through the corps of medical skills. I had hardly learned the various physicians' names as we shook hands and I was briefed in mind-boggling rapidity. Answers were being given which would be adequate for the moment. Later we would be privileged to get acquainted with these men, and they would reveal, in depth, Everett Lee's condition.

"We have drawn off some of the fluid. He is stable for now. We will not know for a while if the blockage causing the buildup of fluid is temporary or permanent. We will learn the answers to your questions as we go along."

That was all I had time to listen to then. Mary Lee would be coming out of the anesthetic soon, and I wanted to be with her. The walk to her room was a long one. I had been on many long, wearisome hikes in the out-of-doors, but this was the most taxing walk I had ever known. On the other end of the twisting, impersonal hall was a person who shared with me all of life's dreams and hopes. She was already weakened by her physical ordeal. How could I break this news to her? What words were there to say that the boy anticipated and born of our love was not normal?

Mary Lee was still asleep. God allowed several minutes for me to sit at the side of her bed. I focused on the one who came into the world's darkness to give it light: "Father, I know you are in this with us. Please give me the words to tell Mary Lee about our baby. Please fill this room with your love."

The walls of the room had seemed to be pressing in, but now they began to recede. The light of God's goodness caused the gloom to lift. A peace

settled upon me that I cannot to this day understand, for which I can only be grateful. Then the
steady breathing from the bed altered, and sheets
rustled.

"How is the baby?" These were her first words.

I held her hand. After pausing, I said, "He has
some problems."

To my surprise, there was no violent emotional
outpouring. God had preceded me, preparing Mary
Lee as he had prepared me. While under anesthesia,
Mary Lee had heard one comment very clearly.
When the baby was born, the doctor had exclaimed,
"Would you look at that!" No doubt this was a
reference to the little fellow's enlarged head. Mary
Lee's memory of the doctor's spontaneous state-
ment provided a warning that all was not well.

I shared with her what the doctor had told me
about Everett Lee. God wanted no dishonesty or
secrets here. We had a time of sweet communion
together. We were not absolved from fear and pain,
but we were released from their potential destruc-
tiveness. God was very near, and we learned, without reluctance, to lean hard upon him.

Before Mary Lee went back to sleep, we entered
into prayer, united in mind and spirit. "Father, if
you want us to raise a child like this, we are will-
ing to do it. If you can trust a boy like this to us,
we will commit him to you to do with as you will.
We will raise him completely to your honor and
glory."

In the days following, we learned much about
this strange-sounding hydrocephalus. And we

learned more about the grace of God. Dr. John Raaf and his assistant Ruby Waterston became "family" to us and to Everett Lee. The other physicians and nurses were very kind and helpful. Of course, Sally Hayes, R.N., Everett Lee's maternal grandmother, was a generous added grace from God. She personally supervised our son's care and interpreted to us the medical jargon bombarding our ears.

We learned that Dr. Raaf was the widely acclaimed dean of neurologists. His quiet strength and unexcelled skill were always a great encouragement to us. On some occasions as many as a dozen doctors sent from other parts of the country and world would follow him into the room. They would listen intently as Dr. Raaf and Mrs. Waterston examined and discussed Everett Lee, learning from this master physician.

On the third day of our son's life, Dr. Raaf confided his diagnosis to me. Together we stood looking at a dripping set of fresh X rays. He pointed out the blockage preventing the cushioning fluid in the brain cavity from taking its normal course back into the bloodstream. Only a few years earlier, there had been no treatment for such a blockage, and the textbook pictures showed children without hope. But an operation had been developed to relieve the pressure. The doctor planned to perform surgery on Everett Lee in two weeks. The purpose of waiting was to allow the baby's strength to build. Meanwhile, fluid would be drained with a needle every other day.

I was startled at the nature of the operation. A shunt—a simple pump—would be installed in Everett Lee's head. Tubes would run from both ends of the shunt. One would lead to the fluid pocket in the brain. The other would run under the surface of Everett Lee's neck, then follow a vein into his heart. This device would complete the normal cycle, returning the excess fluid to circulation in the bloodstream.

I was even more shocked as the doctor pointed back to the X rays. The head on the screen was abnormally large. The doctor outlined the shape of the brain. It was tiny and tear-shaped—about the size of a golf ball. Dr. Raaf said surgery was warranted because of the vitality of Everett Lee's cries and leg movements, but he added, "I don't want to give you unjustified hopes. That brain would usually be considered too small for real intelligence." His candor was matched by compassion and concern.

Once again I had to tell Mary Lee the hard facts. She was preparing to leave the hospital. I was grateful for the remarkable return of strength which God had provided her. With amazing speed she had recuperated from the suffering of the former weekend. However, we felt an ache deep within when we passed through the hospital doors without our baby. We were going home, but we knew that for weeks we would be "visiting" our house, with the hospital as home base.

During the following days, church responsibilities claimed my full attention. Our extended family in the church shared our lives and our needs through that difficult time. We united in prayer, in the uncommon intimacy that only the Spirit of God can create. Together we were learning the joy of complete dependence on God.

On the appointed day, the shunt was successfully installed. Everett Lee, 15 days old, withstood the five-hour surgery very well. However, we were again shocked when the bandages were at last removed. With the fluid drained away, his head took on a grotesque appearance. In the months of his development, the bony structure of his skull had become large enough to contain the excess fluid. Now the bandages came off, revealing a collapsed structure of overlapping bone. But the doctor was unperturbed. He said he would take care of the problem in a few months.

Finally, four weeks after his birth, we brought our brave little fellow home to complete and to bless our family. This baby would become a heavenly gift by his effect on our lives.

We kept his head covered in public for the next five months, until God would provide for his ugliness to be turned into beauty. That transformation had already taken place in our hearts. One day the world would know. But meanwhile, bonnets and hats concealed the sight that might have caused people to gasp. It seemed unfair to him and to the casual observer to reveal that startling head.

We received a poem in a letter shortly after Everett Lee's birth. It challenged and encouraged us.

My Broken Doll

A broken doll was sent to me
   From Heaven up above,
A broken doll to have and hold,
   A broken doll to love.

My joy was turned to sadness,
   My life I thought was done,
I'd hoped the doll I would receive
   Would be a perfect one.

But God does send us varied things,
   He even sent His Son;
Recall the passage in His prayer—
   Thy will, Lord, be done.

God could have sent a perfect doll,
   But our broken one was blessed;
It strengthened my faith and love,
   I hope I've passed my test.

It's strange how that which seemed so sad
   Should be a joy and fun;
I thank God for this priceless gift,
   My broken doll, my son.

                    —Ted Farrell

Mary Lee and I agreed to ask three specific things of God for our "broken doll." These were the deepest longings of our hearts for Everett Lee. We knew in human terms we were asking for the improbable or even the impossible, but we determined to express these longings in faith: "Father, please give Everett Lee a good mind. We ask that he will come to really know you. We pray that his life may bring glory and praise to your holy name."

CHAPTER FOUR

By God's Grace

"DON'T GET your hopes too high," one person said.

Another advised, "Don't expect too much. It would take nothing short of a miracle for him to approach normal life."

Yes, we knew that! The doctors had made it very clear. We were not expecting too much, because we had been instructed to expect nothing. Whatever progress God would help this little boy make would be a bonus. Small or great, it would be a precious gift of God's grace. Our hopes for Everett Lee would have to be written one day at a time.

"Nothing short of a miracle!" All right, but what is a miracle? We knew Jesus Christ had healed the sick. The Scriptures tell us he enabled blind men to see.

When Lazarus was taken ill, the Lord said, "This

. . . is for the glory of God." We didn't know how, but we wanted our lives and Everett Lee's to bring glory to God, too.

A working definition became real to us. Any situation that by its nature or timing would bring glory to God was a miracle. We dared to ask more as God day by day supplied these miracles.

As we held and cared for Everett Lee, we permitted ourselves to think about only one day at a time. Our family learned much as our love deepened for this unattractive baby. Daily we claimed the promise in Philippians 4:19: "My God shall supply all your needs according to His riches in glory by Christ Jesus."

In December God miraculously transformed Everett Lee. Skilled physicians reworked the bony structure of his skull. The bandages came off in time for Christmas. We could scarcely believe it! What a wonderful gift. He had a new head!

It took two operations, 10 days apart, to accomplish the task. Doing half the project at a time, the doctors peeled back Everett Lee's scalp and forehead. After they had sculptured a normal head contour and cut away excess bone, they covered their work by replacing his neatly trimmed scalp and forehead. Suddenly we could see in him family resemblances.

"He has your nose, just like the other kids," Mary Lee remarked.

"His eyes are big and expressive like yours," I replied. "And look! His head is shaped a lot like Fred's."

Kathy found a couple of freckles, "like me," she said.

We were filled with gratitude. God had provided a miracle. For the first time we would take Everett Lee to church with no covering on his head.

Jo Ann observed, "Everyone can look at him now. God has made him pretty."

Soon after Everett Lee's birth, some examiners had expressed questions about his vision. Since babies cannot tell you what they see or don't see, we were urged to have his eyes examined, to find out if the pressure of the prebirth fluid had impaired his vision.

Everett Lee was eight months old when we all loaded into the station wagon to take him to a highly recommended ophthalmologist. We soon learned that the doctor excelled in examining little children. A son of his had been born blind. Perhaps his examination of Everett Lee brought back memories of his own anguish, for at one point it seemed to us that he almost wept.

The doctor drew a chair up close to Mary Lee and me. He leafed through the medical book in his lap and showed us a page with a dozen circles of color. The colors ranged from vivid pink-orange in the upper left corner to blue-white at the bottom right. Very deliberately, he explained that these circles illustrated the full range in condition of optic nerves. The bright color of the healthy optic nerve was pictured in the upper left. The circles graduated downward in declining health, finally illustrating a totally dead nerve in the bottom right photograph. His voice broke slightly as he pointed to the lower right-hand corner.

"Your son has total optic nerve atrophy in both eyes," he said. He explained that pressure from the prebirth fluid had killed these sensitive tissues. Everett Lee's optic nerves were dead.

"How does he follow movement in objects that we pass before him?" we asked, almost in disbelief. "Does this mean he'll never see anything at all?"

The doctor answered our questions as if he were bearing the burden of this news with us. "He may see something. Some persons who have optic nerve atrophy can see light. They can find a lighted window or doorway. It may be so with this baby. If it is, be grateful. As little as it may seem, any vision helps dramatically in mobility."

I don't remember returning to the waiting room for our other children. We were dazed. We had been prepared for a report of some damage—but blindness!

The kids were asking what the doctor had said. They had to be told. "Father, please help me tell Fred, Jo Ann, and Kathy. Please help all of us handle the news that Everett Lee is blind."

We were driving through Portland's city center, but the traffic, buildings, and hurrying people faded. The six of us, including the baby clutched so tightly in his mother's arms, were in a world apart. A grievous sob wrenched from the core of Fred. "You mean he'll never be able to play ball with me?" He was expressing the hurt we all felt. Yes, even this expectation from the heart of a loving brother had to be surrendered to God.

For all of us and for Everett Lee, victory would come—gradually, but in a way that would bring great glory to God. God would supply a significant measure of vision through those dead optic nerves. The doctors would continue to claim that Everett Lee's eyeballs were unable to communicate with his brain. But he would see!

The doctors marveled at this functional miracle. Again and again they sent him on little errands: "Go get my pencil," or "Everett, go to the desk and get my book." They shook their heads in amazement as they tested this miracle boy. Men and women with many years of study in medical science were as elated as we in observing this boy defying the books.

After the first diagnosis, we enrolled him in Oregon School for the Blind. However, it was not necessary for him to be taught braille. Everett Lee's vision certainly was not 20-20, but it progressively improved until he could read large-print books.

He had sung "I see the moon, the moon sees me" for several years. But imagine our rejoicing one night when he made his own observation. It was in another car, but the same select group was present. He inquired, "Mommy, what is that bright round thing up there? Is that the moon?"

In his eagerness to share in the sights others enjoyed, Everett often said he "saw" one object or another. Tonight, however, we knew from the tone of his voice that he had actually seen the moon for the first time. We stopped the car. Again tears were shed, but this time they were tears of joy. "Father, thank you for Everett Lee's unexplainable vision."

We were learning more dependence on God and his goodness. When Everett Lee reached 14 months, another miracle instructed us. The shunt clogged, and Everett Lee was in serious trouble. All symptoms indicated the fluid was building extreme pressure. This little pump had failed before, when his skull was still flexible, so we'd had several hours to observe whether the shunt would clear itself. We could flush it manually and wait to see if it reactivated. However, now Everett Lee's cranial bones had fused. We didn't know this important fact, and we delayed longer than we should have in getting him to the hospital.

Everett Lee was very listless as we admitted him to the emergency room. But we relaxed somewhat, knowing he was under the care of very capable professionals who knew of his medical history. The staff at Good Samaritan Hospital had come to know all of us very well in the last year and a half.

A neurologist treated him in the emergency room. Then the staff settled him into a room directly across from the nurses' station. We slipped out to get a cup of coffee in the hospital cafeteria. The tensions of uncertainty at home, the drive from Woodburn, and the assistance we had provided in emergency-room treatment had combined to exhaust us.

As we were returning, a code-99 call came on the hospital intercom. It was for Everett Lee's room! We ran up the stairs.

A code 99 brings hospital staff with many types of equipment running from every corner of the hospital. We arrived in the middle of the flurry. The head nurse intercepted us before we were able to enter his room. Hospital staff are never sure how family members will respond in a time of crisis. She whisked us into an office across the hall.

Immediately Mary Lee and I joined hands and united in prayer. We knew that our baby was facing death in this critical moment. More calmly than is characteristic of either of us, we again committed this miracle life to God. "Father, he is yours to do with as you please. Whether it be by life or death, we ask only that your name be glorified. Please prepare us further to raise this child of yours, or strengthen us to accept his death."

By my watch, seven minutes had passed since we were seated in that little office. Then, above the other sounds, we heard our baby cry out. The breath of life had been returned!

"Thank you, Father," we breathed.

A nurse who had walked into Everett Lee's room had discovered that he had no vital signs. No blood pressure! No pulse! No breath! The buildup of fluid in his head had turned off his nervous system. Thus the alarm had been broadcast.

Fluid was drained from his head by a needle. Then electroshock was used, along with other stimulation. And he revived!

The hospital staff feared he had suffered permanent brain damage. Brain cells begin to die after four minutes without oxygen, and at least eight minutes had passed for Everett Lee. The doctors warned us to expect some, if not extensive, damage.

Everett Lee was limp and weak the next day. The doctors' fears seemed to be verified. Mary Lee and I prayed throughout our vigil. I moved Everett's passive legs in exercise for many hours during those days. Then he began to regain strength rather quickly. Power returned to his arms and legs. His spunk and wit resurfaced. In a few more days it was clear that he had no apparent brain damage. Once again, heads wagged in amazement.

Everett Lee's brain was a special work of God from the beginning. We were not as surprised as we once might have been by this demonstration of God's special care of that brain.

I later discovered some permanent damage. Everett Lee would wear to the grave the marks of electroshock. The surgical "cut-down," incisions for inserting electrodes in his feet and hands, had left scars. It was as if the one who permanently wears the prints of nails in his hands and feet was marking this little boy.

In various ways we experienced the miracle power of God's grace. He showed us that power by giving us medical technology and dedicated doctors. We saw it revealed in our son's gradual progress, for which there was no scientific explanation. And we saw it in God's intervention to meet our needs in times of crisis. In these three distinct ways, God gave us miracles.

"My Father is omnipotent, and that you can't deny; A God of might and miracles, 'tis written in the sky." Everett Lee would lustily sing John W. Peterson's song.

It took a miracle to put the stars in place.
It took a miracle to hang the world in space.
But when he saved my soul,
Cleansed and made me whole,
It took a miracle of love and grace.

CHAPTER FIVE

Handling a Miracle

As Everett Lee grew, he expressed himself often in song. The songs he loved to sing had
special meaning for our family.

We deliberately tried to fill our home with melody and gospel songs. If our house had only one
electrical appliance, I would prefer it to be a
phonograph or tape deck. We were careful in select-
ing records and tapes, for music fills not only the
interior of a building but also the minds and hearts
of the occupants. Our collection of records and
tapes is a source of delight. Perhaps none of our
other possessions represents as much thoughtful in-
vestment. We have wanted the music to reflect the
"new song" about which David spoke in Psalm 40.

When we first heard Bill and Gloria Gaither's
song, "You're Something Special," we fell in love
with it. Each of us thought it could have been

written about our family and Everett Lee. It certainly expressed how Mary Lee and I looked at our children. Each one was unique and very special to us. We considered it important that they know we loved each of them no less than the latest addition. We were glad this song helped us share these feelings with our kids.

Together we decided to sing this new song for others. We were not and are not a suave, show-business family troupe. Mary Lee accompanied the rest of us on the piano, working hard to master the simplified piano edition and her stage fright. Daddy, who used up his voice back in a college quartet, joined in and coached. The two impishly shy girls and their self-conscious but able teenage brother surrounded Everett Lee. The song was divided to provide each of these special people with a solo part.

The audience for this effort was the Liberty Christian Church in Salem, Oregon. God had directed us to this ministry, allowing Everett Lee to attend the Oregon School for the Blind while living at home. We were encouraged before singing by the appreciative and uncritical spirit of the church. We prayed, "Father, please overcome our fears. May we be used by you to illustrate this happy message to every listener."

God did give remarkable blessing to us and to those who heard. Everett Lee "stole the show." The young man with the awkward gait and eyes betraying visual handicap won every heart. His big smile revealed unabashed joy, and his intense expressiveness gave an extra dimension to the message. Tears dimmed many eyes as we sang:

> When Jesus sent you to us,
> We loved you from the start;
> You were just a bit of sunshine
> From heaven to our hearts.
> Not just another baby
> 'Cause since the world began,
> There's been something very special
> For you in God's plan. That's why . . .
>
> He made you special,
>   You're the only one of your kind,
> God gave you a body
>   And a bright healthy mind;
> He had a special purpose
>   That He wanted you to find,
> So He made you something special,
>   You're the only one of your kind.

Two months later we were asked to sing the song again for the large family camp, Wi-Ne-Ma Week of Missions. Nearly 1300 persons were gathered in tents and camp trailers that August, many of whom had annually seen the progress God was giving our son. Again the Lord gave power to the message as we sang, inspiring that assembly. Many who regularly attend the event continue to consider that moment a highlight. Our simple, unpolished witness in song reached into many hearts.

We understood from the start that Everett Lee

was "especially special," and that we were fortunate to have him as a member of our family. But along with privilege comes responsibility. We knew we would have to allow for his handicaps without falling into the trap of overprotectiveness. If we were to indulge him too much, he might become ungrateful and selfish. Then our other children might feel bitter or resentful toward Everett Lee or us.

Only God could eliminate fears for our young son's welfare, and only God could provide the wisdom we needed for making important decisions. Therefore, we obeyed the instruction in the New Testament letter of James to ask if we lack wisdom: "Father, please guide us in raising Everett Lee as part of our family. Help us make him special, but no more special than Kathy, Jo Ann, and Fred. Make us express our love to him, yet share our love equally. Please show how you want us to handle this miracle."

How did people handle the material of which miracles were made in Jesus' day? Imagine the care the servants must have shown in handling the wine at the wedding feast in Cana of Galilee. And think for a moment about those who watched in amazement when Jesus made an abundant meal for 5000 out of a boy's sack lunch. They must have been awestricken. Yet neither the wedding wine nor the loaves and fishes were hoarded. They were used for the purpose for which they were created.

Principles revealed in these stories from God's Word provided practical wisdom for us in handling our miracle child. If we hoarded our special child away, attempting to protect him, we would deny him the life of service for which he was created.

We found other practical advice in God's Word. "Train up a child in the way he should go, even when he is old he will not depart from it." We claimed this promise from Proverbs 22:6 by expending strenuous effort in training. We had no idea whether Everett Lee would see old age, but we knew he was to be trained in God's way. Since our deepest longing was that he bring glory to God, we would have to apply "the rod of correction" to his special life, too.

The rod? Yes, Proverbs 22:15 says, "Foolishness is bound up in the heart of a child; the rod of discipline will remove it far from him." It was clear that, in spite of his fragile condition, Everett Lee must be handled the same as our other children. We would sometimes administer the rod, always with the grieved and genuine spirit: "I am doing this because I love you." This would be followed by a generous demonstration of sweet comfort like that which God always provides when he chastens us. Everett Lee, too, must know the security and caring love of godly discipline.

We prayed, "Father, help us to treat him like the others as we administer your intended discipline. Let us curb his will to authority, which you have designed to be over him, without breaking his spirit. We are not expert enough to do this, Father. Please do it through us."

Everett Lee proved always sensitive to our will.

He did not outgrow a transparent desire to please his parents and his teachers. Yet he sometimes had to be chastised. With my arm around him, I'd say, "You won't do it again, will you, young man?"

"No, Daddy. I'll never do it again," he would tell me. And he meant it.

In addition to the Scriptures, we had another source of wise counsel in handling this miracle boy. When Everett Lee was 11 months old, Mollie Vlasnic called to ask if she might visit our home. She was the parent counselor for Oregon School for the Blind. For many years she had traveled around the state, bringing encouragement and wisdom to the families of blind children. We were reassured by her compassion and sensitivity.

On her first visit, she taught our son a song: "Hear the sound of the big bass drum. *Boom*, boom, boom, boom; *boom*, boom, boom." Everett learned quickly to pound his stomach with his fist when the "boom, booms" came. For many months he had fun with this verbal game. Words rather than toys became the object of almost all his play for the next four years. Toys were obscure to him, but words were clear.

From her deep well of experience, Miss Mollie told us, "Treat him normally." She urged that we involve him in all our family activities. She recommended caution and sensitivity to his handicaps, but again and again she said, "Introduce him to all normal experiences." We deeply appreciated her counsel.

Our lives would be filled with tension and alertness to Everett Lee's problems for almost a decade. His place of sleep at night or midday was in the room near Mary Lee. Our antennae would always be waving, night and day, at home or away. Never could we be more than an hour and a half's drive from a major medical center. The trips we did take required advance information of hospitals and physicians.

At all times the byword was caution, but we were determined that Everett live as naturally and normally as possible. We wanted him to enjoy an active life. We would not forget his limitations, but neither would we close him in by overprotection. We exercised great care, yet risked his being included in wide-ranging activities. One day he would know he was handicapped. Our goal, however, was that his personality and testimony would not be hampered.

Mary Lee and I dedicated ourselves to training this special little boy, but God could see that Everett Lee was teaching us more than we were teaching him. In Matthew 18 Jesus called a child to him and used that child as a teaching illustration. The Lord was now teaching us with our young son.

CHAPTER SIX

Strong and Brave

"*H*ow tough are you, Everett Lee?"

He would wrinkle up his nose and snort, with a comical expression on his face. Then he'd exclaim, "I'm tough!"

He loved to make people laugh. This little exchange was one of the early ways in which he brought smiles to many. At church or in the hospital halls, people would ask him, "Everett Lee, are you tough today?" Whether he felt chipper or "rotten," he met the question with the same brave response. Immediately he would screw up his nose, huff and puff, and say, "I'm tough!"

He could always count on this antic to bring a chuckle. Inquirers were amused at his silly little dramatization. But they also marveled at this little boy, whose life often hung in fragile balance. With words or thoughts, they replied, "You sure are tough, Everett."

His preschool years were filled with difficulty, as well as with progress. His life revolved around our home, the church, and the hospital. In his own special way, he loved each person in these places, and they returned love to him.

The hospital staff became Everett Lee's buddies. They allowed Mary Lee to sleep in his room during his stays, providing three-way relief. First, she was present to help in surveillance of him. Second, she was comforted by being near her son. Third, Everett was reassured by his mother's presence.

The hospital was "home away from home" to him. After all, the friends in the white dresses were there. Grandma Hayes, who looked in on him every day, was one of them. And there were frequent visits by Grandma and Grandpa Payton, Grandpa Hayes, aunts and uncles, cousins, brother and sisters, and Daddy.

"What color do you think you'll get this time, Everett?"

In pediatrics each room had a brightly colored door. We knew the answer before we asked. "Green, I hope." It had always been his favorite color.

Through those years Everett would be in nearly every room they had. Seldom did he get his wish. There were more of the other colors. But his color preference was specific and permanent, whether for doors or clothing or jelly beans: "Green, please."

When Everett Lee was almost four, his shunt failed. We were not surprised by the decision to replace it with a new one. At one point we had been told these mechanisms lasted an average of 18 months. This little life sustainer, installed when he was 15 days old, had served almost four years, with few interruptions. His condition was poor whenever these stoppages did occur, however.

The doctors decided to replace only the shunt by attaching the new one to the tubes already leading into his brain and heart. This procedure would cause less distress to his nervous system than if they replaced the tubes as well. Though the tubes eventually would be outgrown, the doctors hoped they would last a while longer.

Once again, he rebounded quickly from surgery, but within a few days the physicians knew the device could not function properly with the old set of tubes. We took him back to the hospital just three weeks after the shunt replacement for a second major operation. The complicated back-to-back surgeries caused us some alarm.

With surgery two days past, the little fellow with the bandage-covered head was doing well. It was the Easter season. I had come to the hospital early to take his weary mother to breakfast while he was still sleeping. When we stepped off the elevator on our way back to pediatrics, a familiar voice was ringing out down the hall, half a football field in length.

We learned later that Everett Lee had greeted the first arrivals to his bedside with a spirited song. They set him on the counter of the nurses' station to sing to a wider audience. Our eyes moistened and

our hearts leaped with joy when we saw this scene.
The wide corridor surrounding the station was
filled with nurses, aides, and doctors. Some were the
familiar staff of pediatrics, but there were additional workers from other sections of the hospital. The
clear voice of the bandaged boy, not yet four years
old, was offering more than entertainment. This
song by Rick Backman was his favorite during
those months.

Jesus Is Alive

Verse 1

On that sacred morning called resurrection day
Came a certain woman, Mary was her name.
When she saw her Master
    was missing from the tomb
She turned around and ran away
Straight to the upper room, shouting . . .

Chorus

Jesus is Alive! Jesus is Alive!
He broke the chains of sin and death.
Jesus is Alive!

Verse 2

After His ascension the scriptures do record
The Holy Spirit fell down upon those saints
    in one accord.
And when they went a-preaching
    a great revival came.
And tho' they spoke to many souls
Their message was the same . . .

Verse 3

Christians were tormented by almost everyone,
But they were not defeated.
The church had just begun.
They suffered many beatings
   and some were even killed
For there was one thing they believed
With this their hearts were filled . . .

Verse 4

By faith of millions
   that church is still around
Witnessing for Jesus wherever man is found.
And if we're goin' to make it
   to heaven some glad day
We all must be witnesses
And here is what to say, tell them . . .

Chorus

Jesus is Alive! Jesus is Alive!
He broke the chains of sin and death.
Jesus is Alive!

We were so proud of our special offspring. But mostly we were grateful that Jesus is alive. "Father, thank you for this exciting fact of history. And thank you for showing him to be alive in and through that little angel in the white gown."

Until he was five years old, it seemed that Everett Lee's hair would never grow out. His head was always recently shaved. But God intended to minimize our son's embarrassment from this point onward. Throughout his school days, the hair covering the surgical scars on his head would never be completely shaved again. He would have other difficulties, but the shunt would not require revision.

His vision had improved slightly, but not enough so that he could enjoy toys. He "turned on" appreciation for any toys given him. Then he set them aside. A small cash register and a hammering peg bench, which stimulated other senses, were among the exceptions. We guarded against television addiction, but he loved the children's program Sesame Street. We knew he learned from this show. He listened intently, his eyes focused on the floor.

His motor damage to the right side of his body became more evident as he grew older. It took great effort for him to use his right hand. We encouraged him to exercise that "helping hand" by choosing projects requiring both hands. He tried valiantly, and he did get limited strength in that hand. With a smile he'd slap its wrist and say, "Get busy and help, you lazy hand."

We were accustomed to the deficient hand and the awkward right leg. But when the doctors mentioned "cerebral palsy," they sent arrows of fear into our hearts. They quickly dispelled our dark imaginings. Cerebral palsy is not a disease. It is simply the label attached to brain damage. Everett's cerebral palsy was caused by damage before his birth. Understanding that it was not progressive, we were able to relax. All of that had been committed to the Lord long ago.

God was going to improve our son's ability to walk. Surgery lengthened the tendons in Everett Lee's right ankle and lower leg. Additional operations for hip release helped substantially. He would never be without a pronounced limp, but it would keep him from very few activities.

While he was wearing leg braces, he questioned Mary Lee one day. "Mommy, am I crippled?" We were not sure where he had heard that word. It had not been part of our vocabulary.

"You can walk, can't you?" Mary Lee replied. Agreement was nodded. "Then you are not crippled, are you?"

"No. Then I'm not crippled."

This answer was adequate for the moment. It was like answering a child's question about birth by a simple, "God made you grow in Mommy's tummy." At some time in the future this answer would not be sufficient, but for now it was. It would be some time before Everett Lee realized there was anything he could not do. No, he was not crippled.

Sue Hanks of the Oregon Medical School had designed many exercises to meet Everett's therapy needs. Of all his therapy, Everett liked the Clapper Dappers the least. These aluminum foot-shaped objects, approximately a man's size six, were strapped under his shoes to help his heel-toe gait. We tried to humor him in their use, but they were terribly awkward, noisy, and aggravating—in short, no fun at all.

Just as we began to think about preschool classes for Everett Lee, we learned of a new Montessori kindergarten in neighboring McMinnville. What a coincidence! Through this program God provided a good foundation of encouragement for Everett Lee. Judith Teneau had started the kindergarten in conjunction with Linfield College. Some teachers would have been reluctant to take a student with Everett Lee's limitations. However, she welcomed our little guy with his special needs and treated him the same as the other children.

The school's philosophy was learning by doing. Everett Lee took his turns at washing the group's drinking glasses, and he put his own shoes on and tied the laces himself.

Under the skilled watchfulness of the teacher, he was not endangered by too much or hurt by too little responsibility. He learned near-independence and respect for others.

Mary Lee's mother was close at hand through all of Everett Lee's problems, lending her calm support and deep faith. But when his third major seizure occurred, she was not there. After a rather brief illness, Sally Hayes had gone to her heavenly home from a room in the same hospital where she had worked for 25 years. Her knowledge and comfort had been a tremendous help. God had allowed her to be available through Everett's greatest periods of difficulty.

The seizure that followed her death by six weeks

began very hard. I was not at home when the seizure began, so Yamhill's city policeman drove Mary Lee to meet the Newberg ambulance. An hour and a half elapsed before she arrived with Everett Lee at the hospital. I arrived later, and we spent seven hours with him until the seizure's symptoms subsided.

When Everett Lee recovered from this terrible energy drain, we were given a syringe and medicine to take home. The doctors told us to give him an injection immediately, should another seizure of this type occur.

As we drove toward home with our boy, Mary Lee poured out her heart in prayer. She expressed how deeply she missed the comfort of her mother's presence. Honestly she named her fear of ever having to use the syringe. Then she prayed, "Father, I'll accept your will. But please don't allow Everett Lee and us to endure any more of these seizures. I don't think I can stand it."

Only God knows the limit of our endurance. 1 Corinthians 10:13 promises, "God is faithful, who will not allow you to be tempted beyond what you are able."

We are grateful for the answer our faithful God gave to this prayer. Our little fellow took a daily dosage of medicine, but he never had a similar seizure. We praised God for this victory.

We discovered that Everett means "strong and brave." This boy who had caused many smiles by his "I'm tough" antic was challenged by the descriptive name God had attached to him. He would

say, "My name is Everett. I am strong and brave."
He knew that God was the source of this strength.

"You sure are, young man. You sure are," we
would reply. Sometimes he was stronger and braver
than we.

CHAPTER SEVEN

A
Special
School

EACH YEAR the administration of Oregon
School for the Blind planned two and a half days to
demonstrate their program. They invited parents
of visually handicapped preschoolers to sleep and
eat on campus. Teachers conducted classes for families who were facing problems similar to our own.
We found the fellowship with other parents extremely encouraging. For the Paytons, the annual
events began a love affair with the wonderful staff
of this special learning center.

"I was scared to death!" one young mother exclaimed.

Another woman said, "All those textures drove
me nuts. When I went through those ropes, it was
like being grabbed by a dozen octopuses."

"It seemed like we were in there an hour. And I

thought we had covered a couple of football fields!"
Mary Lee said.

Twenty parents had just passed through the
school "fun house," as the kids called it. We all had
the same reactions, though some of the burly dad-
dies were reluctant to admit having been "scared to
death."

Volunteers from the Lions Club had built this
unusual place for the benefit of the blind children.
It was a basement room approximately 50 by 50
feet, completely closed off in darkness. We parents
were blindfolded and introduced to its various dark,
winding passages.

The room had been carefully planned and constructed to present many obstacles and many sensa-
tions. There were inclines, slats, carpets, corners,
concrete slabs, and slippery surfaces. Heights varied
from adequate for standing to extremely low, requiring even little people to crawl. There were dead
ends and one alleyway from which the only exit
was a ladder. In another area heavy ropes were
hung from the ceiling so tightly that we had to
fight our way through them.

The room also provided different kinds of sounds.
Each step on the ramp beyond the ladder produced
a hollow reverberation. Cymbal-like metal objects
hanging from the roof crashed together as we
passed.

It seemed that we were in the room an hour, and
that we covered a great distance. Yet it was a small
room, and we were there only half an hour. All of
us were both shocked and enlightened by this sen-

sory experience. It made a lasting impression, helping us understand the world in which our children lived. The staff members told us the "fun house" was very important in training the students; I remember thinking that the benefit to parents was perhaps as great.

The O.S.B. campus is ideally located near downtown Salem beside scenic Bush Park. The shadow cast by the towering Salem Memorial Hospital was a comfort to us. The school has its own infirmary, attended by a registered nurse, but the hospital next door provided extra insurance.

The school's specialized facilities had first come to my attention a year before Everett Lee's birth. I was returning to my car after making hospital calls. Then I stopped short, transfixed by what I saw. A young man was running at breakneck speed, back and forth in a dirt rut.

When I moved closer, the picture was suddenly clarified. This young athlete was blind. As he ran, he grasped a handle linked to a guy wire above. He was dashing back and forth, trusting completely in the unseen wire above his head.

This sight portrayed to me the faith we are to have. We also must put our hand out for leadership as we run the course of life. Our guidance is not from a cold, impersonal wire, but from God. His loving and capable hand is extended to us, offering direction above our confusion.

As I watched this boy running with so much enthusiasm, I thought, "What if he let go of the chain? He would immediately be frustrated and defeated by confusion. He would not know where he was going or what was ahead. Probably he would fall headlong over some obstacle or quit running altogether because of fear."

God used that unsighted boy to illustrate eloquently the need for constant faith. I went on my way thankful that God does extend his hand when we have fallen in blindness. He does reach out when we are paralyzed by fear. He longs to lead us through Christ Jesus to excellence in the race of life.

During O.S.B. visitors' days, we parents also watched athletic competitions. I have always liked sports, but Everett Lee and his classmates showed us a whole new dimension of athletics. Their competition was different. Some could run on the full track, and a few would wrestle in the state tournament, but others were physically handicapped. Yet each was made to feel important

The field days to which families were invited annually were an inspiration. Jo Ann and Kathy were thrilled at being asked to help. They assisted the staff in seeing that every child was challenged and none was belittled. Everyone was a winner as the day proceeded. There were piggyback races, with older kids carrying the younger. Contests such as Cracker-Doodle permitted the more handicapped to compete. It was hilarious to watch the children chewing generously peanut-buttered crackers and then trying to whistle "Yankee Doodle."

The highlight, however, was the Balloon Belly Shuffle. Each pair of contestants, with their hands behind their backs, pressed a water-filled balloon between their stomachs and tried to race to a line and back without dropping or breaking the balloon. The school principal, Neil Kliewer, always joined this competition, and he was the star of the event. For all these activities, the staff provided a radio-like blow-by-blow description of progress. The kids constantly asked, "How is Mr. K. doing?" And when the balloon of the beloved Mr. K. broke, a loud cheer went up.

The day concluded with an impressive awards assembly in the school auditorium. Ribbons were presented to winners of the day's races. There were also citations for achievements in the regular physical education classes.

In this same auditorium, the classes brought carefully rehearsed programs twice a year. They were always entertaining, but at some point I always choked up, watching those little folks perform for an audience they could not see.

"Father, thank you for these blessed little children. Please reward them for the efforts they are making far beyond my applause or the tiny awards. And may their instructors receive from you the awards they so richly deserve for their beautiful ministry."

Everett Lee had been a student for only a year when Mary Lee and I were included in a special school activity. The older children and the staff members and their families were attending a dress rehearsal of the *Helen Keller Story* at a theater near the school, before the production opened to the general public. The director, anticipating the added impact a talented blind girl would have, cast a young O.S.B. student for the part of Helen Keller.

The moving story of the deaf-blind child and those who travailed with her to victory was never more powerfully portrayed. The story was very familiar to this audience, most of whom could not see, and they hung on every word. Mary Lee and I observed the observers almost as much as we watched the play. The story of a courageous blind girl, being played by a blind girl, was itself inspiring. But the rapt attention of this special audience added goose bumps to my goose bumps.

"Thank you, Father, for this wonderful group of which Everett Lee is a part. And thank you for using them to remind us that blind is beautiful, too."

CHAPTER EIGHT

Special Teachers

"OH NO, not you!" he moaned.

We had just settled into the restaurant booth with a family of close friends for dessert after a football game. The final score had gone our way, and everyone's spirit reflected it.

"Oh no," he continued. Each time he repeated it, he turned the volume up a notch until finally the adults halted their busy conversation.

Then we saw the object of his exclamation. Everett Lee had spotted one of his teachers. We tried to hush Everett, but we might as well have tried to "shush" a rooster at dawn.

"Oh no, not you!" he repeated in delight.

We were embarrassed. It was clear to us that he was teasing, but we were not sure that the Friday night restaurant crowd would understand.

Mrs. Wentzel took it very well. By working

closely with Everett Lee, she had come to understand this style of teasing as his highest form of compliment. His "Oh no" was really a squeal of joy at seeing someone he especially liked.

His teachers at O.S.B. were certainly in that category. From his early days at the school, Arloene Summers was Everett Lee's special teacher. She had read the reports in his files dating back to birth. But reports of optic nerve atrophy and the early description of poor learning capacity did not discourage her. She saw in Everett a little boy with special circumstances who had been entrusted to her. The plan she implemented was the "accentuate the positive and eliminate the negative" song theme. With the finest balance of sternness and tenderness that I have seen, she introduced this boy to miraculous progress.

We were surprised at the news that Everett Lee would not be taught braille. He started bringing little cards home from school with him—reading cards! The front card in the rubber-banded pack bore the teacher's instructions to me: "If he can read this set to Dad, Everett will receive three smiling faces." Below was a line for my signature when the assignment was completed. Yes, he was learning to read, and he was actually seeing those large, hand-written words!

You can bet that Dad was very happy to sit down and act as an extension of the teacher. Smiling faces were little incentives paying big dividends. Whenever a child had accumulated 10 smiling faces, he or she earned one "peak." On Friday afternoons the students would choose peaks from a box of little goodies that Mrs. Summers kept in her desk. These treasures were offered to reward diligence. Mary Lee and I smiled when Everett brought home an ugly rubber spider and a shrill whistle. We saw his pride in presenting them to us. He truly enjoyed learning, and he stood nine feet tall in his accomplishments.

At one point we seriously discussed not teaching Everett Lee to write. Mrs. Summers didn't want him to become frustrated. His "good" left hand was shaky, and his first efforts to print were painfully difficult. She assured us that he could complete schooling by doing lessons on a dictaphone. We agreed that this was a better alternative than causing him to despair over his inability to write.

Again, God intended to glorify his name. No school papers brought Everett more pleasure than those he wrote himself. Math and spelling worksheets were the first samplings of these efforts. Although they may not have compared with the legible printing of many second graders, those painstakingly scrawled letters were a great achievement. Writing was never easy, but Mrs. Summers' patience and Everett's stubborn hard work brought success.

Everett's classroom guide from first grade on was this same teacher. There were no moves each year to a different class. Mrs. Summers was intent upon seeing him equipped to enter the regular school system. The pupil and his teacher had a very special relationship. During one of his hospital stays, she sent him a get-well card on which she wrote, "You have a freckle dancing all over your nose just begging for a kiss."

From his bed, Everett Lee broke into laughter. "That's Mrs. Summers!" he said.

At school, when she made that statement, she would kiss the offending freckle. He would always respond by breaking up in a flood of giggles.

Sharing "very special teacher" status was the handwork instructor Gen Bridges. Mrs. S. and Mrs. B. worked together marvelously. As soon as three smiling faces were given on a piece of work, Everett would receive the maximum reward. Mrs. S. would send him to Mrs. B. for a smack on the cheek and a swat on the bottom!

Mrs. Bridges guides all children in the school to produce fine objects with their own hands. Our son made things we thought impossible: driftwood patio strings, ornamental candles, resin-disc wind chimes, glazed pottery, breadboards, berry scoops, and a decorative small chair. Supervised by this incredibly patient and artistic woman, he mastered those inefficient hands. We happened into the shop room one day as he was nailing the roof onto a birdhouse. We were amazed. In spite of his clumsy hands and poor vision, he controlled the vise, hammer, nails, and wood successfully.

All year long the children labored toward a public open-house sale. Their crafts were of commercial quality, and when the three-day event ended, nearly every object had been sold. The youngsters earned half the price on all items. The other half went toward the purchase of materials. Their satisfaction and pride in their excellent work was the most valuable benefit, but it was fun to see them receive the envelopes with the carefully accounted cash from their sales. This was the only money most of them would earn all year.

The school sponsored many field trips. Often Mary Lee, Jo Ann, and Kathy were included—extra hands were needed to care for the group. Several times the students went to the beach to gather driftwood for crafts. They went on a two-day retreat, and they made an out-of-state visit to Mary Hill Museum.

On one trip a Washington State patrolman drove up as Everett Lee was helping crank up the tent trailer. Before others could speak, Everett said, "They make me work so hard."

As the officer was about to reply, Mrs. Bridges asked, "Yes, is child labor against the law in this state?"

The field trips were exciting and very important stimuli for these children. The instructors carefully provided a variety of experiences to expand their understanding. On some occasions the students were asked to appear at the state capital building or sing in the lobby of a bank. Wherever they went, they expanded people's understanding.

On a trip to the zoo, our son got more than he bargained for. The kids were assisted in getting close enough to touch the animals. They were surrounding a young elephant when she aimed her trunk at Everett Lee and "whuffed." Instantly he backed up, protesting: "Mrs. Summers, that elephant blew her nose on me!"

All the kids and staff had a good laugh from his objection. These classmates were a very special fraternity, and their sighted guides were part of it.

Everett's class consisted of 10 children, very different but deeply bonded in friendship. They learned to make allowances for each other's deficiencies as they learned to handle their own. They shared the hard reality of handicaps, but they shared great fun, as well.

Once our son came home reporting that he was running for student body office. We were pleased when he later reported his election to the position.

"What does School Fire Chief of the Year do?" we asked.

He patiently explained to his ignorant parents the elaborate duties of fire chief. Once a month he was to appoint the day for the all-school fire drill. The honor accorded our young man was very significant, and he did not take the office lightly.

Mrs. Bridges reported another example of Everett Lee's leadership:

> Every time a dead bird or other small animal was found, the children always insisted upon a funeral. They wanted a proper burial.
>
> One day we found that our pet horned toad had expired. Travis started crying. Everyone was sad. They asked if we could have a funeral during class. I said, "All right, but we will need someone to be in charge of the service."

Everett cleared his throat, stood up tall, and announced, "I'll be happy to do it. I'm going to be a preacher when I grow up!"

He did a beautiful job. Flowers covered the grave; there was singing and a short sermon.

Honor must be given where honor is due. All of the excellent staff and special classmates of Oregon School for the Blind are on our commendation list. Each one gave so much assistance and added so much joy to our son's life. "Thank you" seems pitifully inadequate to express our gratitude.

"Father, thank you for providing Everett Lee with these specialists. Please confirm to them that their devoted efforts were not wasted on him. And, Father, thank you for the miracle gift of his capacity to learn."

CHAPTER NINE

Leader and Friend

We ARE GRATEFUL beyond words for God's goodness in Everett Lee's education. At the same time, we are possibly more grateful for what God taught us through our son.

The Lord intends every child to instruct his family. In teaching the disciples, Jesus "set a child in the middle of them" to illustrate important truth. He said, "Suffer the little children to come unto me, and forbid them not: for of such is the kingdom of heaven" (KJV). On another occasion he explained, "Unless you become like children, you shall not enter the kingdom of heaven."

Each baby entering a family teaches a larger dimension of love to Mom and Dad. Family members learn greater unselfishness. They come to understand dependence through ministering to the needs of a little child. Sisters and brothers, right along with Mom and Dad, grow in love and patience as they do what is needed for the one who cannot do for himself. The beauty of human personality before it learns deceit and distrust is witnessed only in "transparent" little ones.

God wants to teach lessons of love and unselfishness with all children, but he may use a handicapped child to teach these lessons in greater depth. Having a baby with special needs is like having title to a rocky and arid piece of property under which is a vein of gold. The wealth will not come with ease, but God intends the "broken doll" to be an enriching gift.

Fred came home from junior high one day with news, "I was sent to the vice-principal's office this afternoon."

Having had some similar experiences as a teenager, I was anxious to hear the reason.

"I knocked a boy down in the locker room," he reported.

Our family has been trained in the old-fashioned "get a whipping at school, get another at home" philosophy. We want to support the authorities. We were surprised to learn that Fred had not been suspended and no punitive action had been taken. It made sense when he explained the rest of the story.

The previous night our family had gone to a basketball game. Fred was on the team. Everett Lee, then five, was with us. Throughout the game he joined in the cheers, about one beat late in the cadence, as usual. Then, as the game concluded, he jumped to the floor and, in his typical awkward fashion, ran to Fred. He wrapped his arms around his brother's legs in a big hug. This was the normal exuberance he expressed at such times. Fred patted him on the shoulder and then hurried on to the shower room.

The next day a bully attempted to get the best of Fred. The whole class of boys was dressing for gym. When Fred refused to cave in to this boy's attempts to humiliate him, the adolescent made another attempt to shame our oldest son, calling for the attention of all the others. "Hey, did you guys see Fred's little brother at the game last night? He's a dumb retardo," the boy sneered.

Hardly were the words out of his mouth when Fred cleared a bench, crossed the room, and planted a haymaker on his chin. The teacher stepped into the area just in time to see a room full of wide-eyed boys. The biggest of them all was on the floor, his nose bleeding and his eyes filled with tears. Standing over him was Fred.

After hearing the full account verified by the other boys, the administrator decided Fred's course of action had fit the situation. We warned Fred against fighting, but it was impossible to conceal our tone of congratulations.

Our family was learning deeper sensitivity for the crippled and deformed. These special people for whom so few have time or concern are seen differently through better-instructed eyes. Fred's zeal in defending his brother against an ugly attack was

73

only a symptom of what had become more obvious in other ways.

It has been said, "He jests at scars who never felt a wound." Everett Lee's family felt some wounds. Some of them were inflicted with words. But the Lord led us away from reacting violently. All of us have come to pity the sad persons who show such unkindness and insensitivity. They are the unfortunate and misled ones.

We are still learning how God keeps his promises. Romans 8:28 tells us that God will bring good as the outcome of all things. We have learned that this good outcome is discovered only by those who are named in the second half of the verse: those who trust and love God in all circumstances. God gave our family more blessings as we trusted him more.

"Father, thank you for the extraordinary opportunities our children bring. Please lead us to the rich gold you intend for us beneath the surface. And, Father, forgive us when our temporal wishes make us ungrateful and at cross-purposes with your will."

A deep sense of friendship was one of the important things Everett Lee taught us. Ministers are advised to be friendly in general, but they are also cautioned to avoid favoritism or cliquishness. As a result, many pastors find it hard to drop a curtain of trained tactfulness. Being a real friend to anyone is difficult because of the quest after friendliness toward everyone.

God broke through this cloudy curtain with the

bright sunshine of our little son. Everett Lee combined friendliness for everyone with in-depth friendship for many. He never saw a stranger, only friends he hadn't met yet.

On the sidewalk in front of our house in Yamhill he met Larry and Judy Parmley, and he launched us into a lasting friendship with this young couple. "Hi! My name is Everett Lee Payton. What's yours?" Barely allowing time for a response, he continued, "What are you doing? I'm unloading groceries for my mom."

The Parmleys had just moved to the little country town and were on a get-acquainted walk. I first met them several days later when they came to our church services. In a short while these believers in Jesus Christ became a part of the church family. Their friendship has brought great joy to the Paytons.

Years later Judy asked me, "Do you know why we came to visit the church that first Sunday?"

"No, I don't," was my honest reply.

She and Larry related the incident of Everett Lee's unabashed friendliness. Not till then did we know that this boy with the obvious handicaps had provoked this happy relationship. God brought us together by our son's genuine and uninhibited search for friends.

Everett Lee had a knack for remembering the special moments or comments that bind people together. Fun times were enjoyed over and over because he recalled them often.

Once Carl and Virginia Hemminger invited us

for a dinner. They asked me to preside over services for a chicken who had "passed away." Every morsel of the "chicken funeral" was savored by us all. The mashed potatoes were Everett's favorite. He ate a plateful of them and sampled everything else.

As the dishes were being removed from the table, Carl asked Everett if he'd enjoyed the dinner. Mimicking a television commercial, he replied with great expressiveness, "I can't believe I ate the whole thing." Then he threw in the TV response: "You ate it, Ralph." The house shook with our laughter.

Several weeks later there was an all-church pot-luck dinner featuring a wonderful selection of farmhouse recipes. After we'd all gorged ourselves, Carl called out from across the room, "Did you get enough to eat, Everett?"

With no prompting, Everett Lee pushed back his chair and stood. His eyes looked toward the end of his nose, betraying his inability to see the questioner. Yet clearly recognizing the voice, he replied, grinning from ear to ear, "I can't believe I ate the whole thing?"

The building practically came down, and the fun of friendship was forever welded between this young man and "the Hem-ming-gers," as he called them. He never forgot the joy of the dinner at their house.

Elmer and Jane Aline were among Everett Lee's closest adult friends. They had followed his progress and were very encouraging from the day of his birth. When he reached six, they gave a birthday party for him at a pizza parlor. Elmer and Jane and all our family had such a good time together that this event became a tradition.

Everett's appetite was adequate, but he was never a big eater. Even with foods he especially liked, he was satisfied with a moderate quantity. But each year that birthday party was the exception. You would have thought this little man had been locked in a closet and starved all year. He devoured the pizza, not at all distracted by the crowded surroundings or the loud player piano. He seemed to know that his ravenous appetite at this celebration sparked joy. His enthusiasm was a contribution he happily made to this friendship. His exaggerated appetite told Elmer and Jane what a boy could not say.

One of the lessons his life taught us was a "how to." Everett Lee showed us all, especially Mom and Dad, how to invest in special friendships. He lifted high a standard in the importance placed upon friends and family.

"Father, thank you for helping us see, through Everett, that friends are truly special gifts. Please lead us further from friendliness in general into your gift of companionship."

CHAPTER TEN

Thanksgiving Living

"*That was* a good sermon, Daddy!"

Others sometimes make this comment as a benign kind of flattery. Everett Lee made it out of very real appreciation. This little boy who desired to become a preacher loved every effort in the name of Christ. If all members in each church were as uncritical and "Colossians 3:17-ish" as he, revival would sweep the land. "And whatsoever ye do in word or deed, do all in the name of the Lord Jesus, giving thanks to God and the Father by him" (KJV).

Our family committed to memory this verse and another that points to the importance of thanksgiving. 1 Thessalonians 5:18 tells us, "In every thing give thanks: for this is the will of God in Christ Jesus concerning you" (KJV).

Many who want the happiness found only in the

will of God miss this command. God's will for us begins with rejoicing as we receive the gifts of forgiveness and new life through Jesus Christ. Then he wants us to live all of life in joy-filled orbit around this hub of gratitude.

We have found a key to a happier life in Christ. It is learning to give thanks in circumstances for which we are not yet thankful. By doing so, we step above our natural emotions to see the situation from God's point of view. He shows us a vision of victory, which can be ours by his power. Then, as we trust him for that victory, change takes place. Satan's design to defeat and embitter us is overcome. As James 1:2 says, the trial can be embraced as a friend. God wants us to live out our testimony in victory over trials.

Everett Lee showed the way for us in thankfulness. We all memorized the verse in Colossians, but he lived it.

One incident in particular stands out clearly in my mind. We had just made a rushed trip to the hospital. At the ambulance entrance, I quickly relieved Mary Lee of the good-sized boy she held. Through the electric-eye double doors, we dashed to the emergency-room desk. Then I held Everett Lee in my arms while the nurses made urgent calls to the resident neurologist and to Dr. Raaf.

Everett was hardly conscious. Shunt failure was causing pressure to intensify in his head. He was very limp. Suddenly the illness triggered his gag mechanism, and he vomited down my back. This aroused him momentarily. He struggled to talk.

"Daddy, I'm sorry I threw up on you," he said with difficulty.

I nearly sobbed at this expression of my son's inner spirit. Certainly he had tried to prevent this incident, but, desperately sick, he could not. Grateful for the care being given, his thoughts were not of himself. Instead he was sorry for the unpleasantness he had caused me.

In a moment he had rebuked many of my wrong attitudes, while showing the beauty of godly ones. This incident prompted much self-scrutiny. Each time I remember his words, I am grieved at my impatience or unkindness when things are not going well.

Another way Everett expressed gratitude was his appreciation for little, simple things. Our family has never been flush with money. This certainly was true in the avalanche of medical expenses. But God has used this veiled blessing to shape gratitude in all of our family for simple things.

Again, Everett Lee led our little band in enjoyment and thanks for any gesture of kindness. Many of us show joy only in the biggest or most expensive gifts we receive. This boy never learned degrees of thankfulness based on those measurements.

People showered this special young man with affection in many wonderful ways. He always responded beyond expectation. Pinkie may be the best example. Perhaps of all the things given to him in his nine years, Pinkie was the most beloved.

Wilma Fahey, from our church family, knit a pink pig for Everett Lee. This small stuffed animal was his bedtime delight. After his prayers, Mary Lee would tuck him into bed each night. The pillows or sheets were unimportant compared to the companion cradled under his arm. The labor and love Pinkie represented never ceased to mean much to him.

He seemed to prefer simple things to the biggest or the best. Most of us respond to the size or cost of generosity. He responded to the thoughtfulness underlying the gesture.

Each day he needed much help. His training gave him a healthy attitude of independence. Still, his diligent efforts in many tasks were frustrated by weakness in one hand and limited dexterity in the other. He always needed help in securing snaps, brushing teeth, tying shoes, ascending or descending stairs. A large burden fell on the young shoulders of his two sisters and brother.

But his ever-present gratitude kept this work from being resented. "Thank you very much" or "Thank you, Jo, Jo," he would say. As they readied him for school, he'd comment, "I love you for helping me." Because of his appreciation, they were able to accept the responsibility, and they grew stronger by their efforts.

"Father, thank you for showing us how attractive a grateful spirit is to human eyes and to yours. Please lead us by the blueprint of Colossians 3:17 and Everett's example to give thanks in all things."

Everett Lee's improving health brought a day with much excitement. We had always been compelled to have his bed beside our own. For six years

Mary Lee had slept with the fabled one eye open. Her restless nights were added to the hectic pace of our church-centered lives. The stamina which God supplied her causes me to marvel.

Now Everett had progressed and stabilized, and we could move his bed out of our room. The room which became his was just beyond our bedroom door. Measuring six feet by nine, it had been designed as a utility area, and it had one window and four doors. The wall decorations consisted of faucets, a drain pipe for a washer, and a vent for a dryer. A peculiar room, but it was his! He had his own cowboy bedspread and a shelf for Pinkie.

For weeks every guest was met at our front door with: "Did you know I have my very own bedroom? Would you like to see it?" With great pride Everett escorted the guest to his room. We were a bit embarrassed to have others view this cramped spot. However, he was not to be denied that privilege.

This tour meant more to him than some guests realized. He was proud and thankful for the growth and health God was providing. More than the room, it was the goodness of our God that was on display. His "very own bedroom" symbolized God's care.

Mary Lee and I were very much aware that God was revealing his loving kindness in our home. We wanted this witness to extend beyond the walls of our house. Out of his own thanksgiving, Everett Lee wanted to share this testimony, too.

One night Mary Lee and I went to nearby Albany to a gathering of several churches. A quartet sang a song that was new to us. We were moved by the happy truth it expressed about the perfection all will know in heaven. We both wanted our family to learn this song.

Mary Lee purchased the sheet music. One afternoon she was practicing on our upright piano. Concentrating on learning the words, she quietly sang as she played. She didn't realize Everett Lee was listening intently off to one side.

Suddenly he walked over to the piano. Tugging hard at her arm, he said, "Mommy! Mommy! Does that mean I won't be crippled in heaven?" Hope welled up within him. "Is that true? Do you mean, Mommy, that I won't be blind when I get to heaven?"

"It is true," she confirmed. Somehow we had never discussed this good news with Everett Lee.

A broad smile broke out on his face. He probably didn't see the tears in our eyes. Completely confident in this new information, he said, "That's really neat. I won't be crippled when I see Jesus."

The song is by Ray Overholt. Everett Lee embraced completely the truth it expresses. Based on the promises of God, it tells an important part of our faith, as well.

Hallelujah Square

I saw a blind man tapping along,
Losing his way as he passed through the throng;
Tears filled my eyes, I said,
  "Friend you can't see."
With a smile on his face, he replied to me.

I'll see all my friends in Hallelujah Square,
What a wonderful time we'll all have up there;
We'll sing and praise Jesus, His glory to share,
And you'll not see one blind man
 in Hallelujah Square.

Now I saw a cripple dragging his feet,
He couldn't walk like we do down the street;
I said, "My friend I feel sorry for you,"
But he said, "Up in heaven
 I'll walk just like you."

I'll see all my friends in Hallelujah Square,
What a wonderful time we'll all have up there;
We'll sing and praise Jesus, His glory to share,
And you'll not see one cripple
 in Hallelujah Square.

Now I saw an old man, gasping for breath,
Soon he'd be gone as his eyes closed in death;
He looked at me and said, "Boy, don't be so blue,
I'm going up to heaven, how about you?"

I'll see all my friends in Hallelujah Square,
What a wonderful time we'll all have up there;
We'll sing and praise Jesus, His glory to share,
And we'll all live forever in Hallelujah Square.

CHAPTER ELEVEN

Fun to Live With

"ARE YOU fun to live with?" This provocative question was the focus of a seminar I attended. It has been my privilege to profit from a number of educational seminars, but few were of more practical help than the one in which this opening question was raised. All relationships benefit when people care enough to bring enjoyment to others.

Everett Lee was fun to live with! He consistently desired to bring happiness to those around him. When he was feeling good, he planted seeds for smiles and reaped a hundredfold. Even in his many times of illness and pain, he illustrated God's truth declared in Proverbs 17:22: "A joyful heart is good medicine." That prescription was a gift from God. Everett gladly took it in large dosage and gave it in even greater measure.

Part of the laughter he brought was unintentional. There were times when the fun bordered on embarrassment—for his family, that is, never for him. He did what came naturally, free from sophistication and embarrassment. When others laughed in delight, our family joined in. Often this was because there was no time or place for the "more proper" ones of us to hide.

For his third Christmas season, we waited in a long line for Everett Lee to see Santa Claus. We never gave our children illusions about a real St. Nick, but seeing Santa was always fun.

This department store had cleverly provided for the children's voices to be broadcast as they told Santa their Christmas wishes. A microphone was concealed under Santa's beard. Parents would place their boy or girl on the costumed lap and then retreat to the spot where the speaker would convey the tot's wishes. The waiting crowd enjoyed this spectacle with each family.

Deep ho-ho-hos were highlighted by flashbulbs. A sweet voice timidly relating a list of hopes would come over the speaker. The parents would then step up and take the smiling child from the Santa's lap. The next ho-ho-ho would sound just as the candy cane gift reached the previous child's mouth.

The crowd behind us was large when our turn finally came. We took Everett Lee forward and then returned to the place in front of the speaker. The kindly gentleman had barely uttered the words, "And what do you want for Christmas?" In lightning quick response, Everett reached out and relieved Santa of his beard! The ho-ho-hos were replaced by howls from the onlooking crowd. Santa turned a shade of red that nearly matched his suit.

Jo Ann and Kathy ran like deer. We didn't see them again until we reached the parking lot. When the car doors slammed shut, we just looked at each other. Then it was our turn to howl in laughter.

Another of these unplanned episodes came in a gospel-music concert. Fred was singing in a fine choral group known as the Sounds of Truth. The concert was given on a Sunday evening in a rather formal church. The leader drew a fine performance from the talented kids, and the selection of songs exalted Jesus Christ.

One number of comic relief was included midway. To introduce it, several of the ensemble members spoke. They dramatically declared the great discouragements facing young moderns: population explosion, shortages of food and fuel, and threat of nuclear holocaust. Priscilla Miller, an attractive high school junior, declared, with feigned weeping, "I'll probably never even be able to get married!" (Sob.) "Nobody will be left to marry me!" (Sob.)

Everett Lee had been listening very carefully. Priscilla was a neighbor to us and a friend of his. He did not realize the students were acting, and the smiles in the audience were invisible to him. Priscilla sounded desperate and hurt. Consequently, before any preventive action could be taken, he stood and declared, "I'll marry you, Priscilla!"

Gales of laughter filled the room. The ensemble

briefly lost their composure. We laughed, too. What else could we do? So did Everett Lee. But everyone, including Priscilla, knew that he had been completely sincere. From a genuine and spontaneous desire to comfort, he had offered to marry her.

Any gathering had an extra element of excitement or fun when it included Everett. If he happened to miss an event at church, at school, or with our family, many commented. "Where is Everett Lee today?" "We sure do miss that little fellow when he's not here." They were noting by his absence the enthusiastic good humor injected by his presence. More often than not, this humor was intentional. Though it seemed to come naturally, this boy worked at creating cheer. It was important to him.

At one point Everett learned the popular song "Hello Dolly" for a school program. Six months later he turned it to special advantage.

The families of Mary Lee and her two sisters came together annually to view Christmas movies, and it has been my responsibility to take the eight-millimeter family record each year. People were always slightly irked by the bright light in their faces, and the mechanics of running and rewinding a dozen 50-foot reels were tedious. All this, however, was accepted in good spirit. Everyone was pleased to have the antics and growth in the families regularly recorded in home movies.

All the Christmas films were strangely similar. The trees, the ornaments, the wrappings, and the cast were basically the same. Only the sizes and shapes of the eight cousins changed significantly. The assembly commented on a new member added to the cast in a certain year. And a reverent hush fell over the group when a now-absent member appeared briefly on the screen.

Large 30-inch-long red stockings had a starring role in the pictures. Mary Lee's sister Joan had made them seven years earlier. Each film from those seven years showed the eight kids holding their full stockings. The impact of this sight began to build after five repeats. On their sixth appearance someone said, "There are the stockings again!"

"I don't know what we'd do without those stockings," Sharon Ann, the third sister, said. All the youngsters nodded their agreement.

These big red containers were about to be shown for the seventh time. All of us were watching for them. Suddenly, there they were, "hung with care," in all their splendor.

Everett Lee, seated directly in front of the screen, had been straining to see what the rest of us were seeing. Now, before anyone else could speak, he broke into full-voice song. "Hello, stockings. Well, hello, stockings. It's so good to see you back where you belong. You're looking swell, stockings, and I can tell, stockings . . . you're still going strong!"

This cleverness prompted a big laugh. We marveled at Everett's quick wit.

Family, friends, and strangers enjoyed that wit.

It was not saved for big occasions, but was spent freely anywhere.

After dinner at the home of our friends Ralph and Bobbie Hewett, Everett Lee was singing from a book taken off the piano. He abruptly paused, exclaiming, "That doesn't sound right!"

Bobbie turned to him and replied, "Well, of course not! Your book is upside down."

He changed it, and with a smile began to sing again. A moment later he stopped and said, "It did help, Bobbie!"

Among the skills in fun which Everett especially developed was teasing. Some people warn against teasing. I agree when it is a method of having fun at someone else's expense. But for Everett Lee, teasing was a special game played with friends who shared his inside information. The tease was a toy which didn't have to be seen to be enjoyed.

"Daddy, come look!" he cried.

I knew exactly what that giggly invitation from our bedroom signaled. Months before, he had told me that he was going to sleep in my bed. I immediately coined a grave threat. "Young man, if I catch you in *my* bed, I'll rub my whiskers on you!" This was one of the strange forms of torture he loved.

Another time the threatened violence would take the form, "If you don't get yourself out of *my* bed, I'm going to dunk you in the ocean." He would then relish the approach of our next beach trip.

Now again from the bedroom it was, "Daddy, come look!"

I peered around the door. There he was under the covers, writhing with glee.

"What do you think you're doing in *my* bed?" I asked in the usual pretense of pain. Then there followed several minutes of feigned anguish. The more dramatic my dismay, the more enthusiastic his giggling.

Similar to the bedroom scene was the little-fork routine. O.S.B. students are trained to set tables, and eventually they perform the task more expertly than sighted folks. Measuring every distance with their hands, they make precisely correct placements of plates and all utensils. Although Everett could get the job done, he was sloppier at it than most of his classmates. His limited vision made him impatient with the slow measurements.

Several months earlier, I had expressed a strong preference for full-sized forks. Apparently my emphasis of this was memorable.

Whenever it was Everett's turn to set the table, we all anticipated what would precede the prayer of thanks. The one little fork buried at the bottom of our utensil drawer would turn up. Searching hands would manage to find it, then conceal it under the edge of my plate or partially cover it with my napkin. Everett would sit awaiting the reaction as inconspicuously as possible while Dad came to the table.

"Where did this thing come from? Who gave me this little fork?" my script read.

He would cover his mouth with his hand in an attempt to hide the flow of giggles. Still breaking up, he would push back his chair as I called for a "real" fork. As soon as the little prop in this play had been retrieved and replaced by the preferred style, we were ready to pray, thanking the Lord for all of his blessings to us. Along with the audible prayer naming the food and events of the day was another: "Father, thank you for the laughter in Everett Lee's life. Thank you for the fun he has brought into our home and for the sweet relief from tensions. Please help me to be fun to live with, too."

CHAPTER TWELVE

Unlimited Service

THE SUNDAY-EVENING SERVICE had just concluded, and the congregation moved slowly out of the warm building to linger in conversation on the lawns. The stately white church house glowed in the light of the setting sun. Sheep and cattle could be seen grazing to the west. A cooling breeze from the Pacific swept down from the mountains.

Enjoying leisurely conversation, families gradually moved toward their cars. People who are in the prime of family life, surrounded by children, cannot know the loneliness others sometimes feel. Even in such a serene setting, there are disquieting times. A couple recalls how, long ago, their little ones surrounded them. An individual walks to the car in which she will make her way home alone.

On this night Fern Ripple was lonely. Her vivacious spirit and faith regularly encouraged the congregation and minister, but now she dreaded the drive home alone. No one else knew her feelings, nor did they need to know. The Lord would see her through as he had so many times before.

Everett Lee was always more sensitive to spirit than to scenery. The moment of her departure was unnoticed by anyone but him. He sensed her need as folks began to scatter in the fading light. Making his way to her, this five-year-old said, "You're here all alone, aren't you? I'll ride as far as my house with you, and that will help."

Our house was 60 paces from where they stood! But this little fellow wanted to do what he could to help. The hurts he had felt so often were of a different nature, but through them God made him alert to the hurts and needs of others.

In the sweetness of her own understanding, Mrs. Ripple opened the car door. She helped Everett in and then drove the width of the church yard and across the driveway. Stopping in front of the Paytons' house, she walked around and assisted him out of the car. With a warm embrace, she said, "Thank you, Everett. It certainly did help!"

He taught our family what it is to be sensitive to people's needs. Mrs. Summers reported that he instructed the O.S.B. faculty and students by this concern for others. She told me, "That boy has made me a believer in ESP! He just seems to know if you have special needs. Then he goes right to work to cheer you up."

We knew that Everett's "ESP" was a gift from God. It made us very thankful that this miracle life was noted as being extraordinary. The praise and honor could only be given back to the Lord.

In Everett's third year at the school, the blind children "kidnapped" Ralph Williamson. Ralph for many years had been a benefactor to these kids in a number of ways. He is a paraplegic whose rock shop and jewelry-making school are run from a wheelchair. One day in their specially equipped bus, Everett Lee's class dropped in without warning to take Ralph to an ice-cream parlor.

This treat was met with enthusiasm. Soon the bus pulled up and unloaded its cargo of special people. The hour had been planned so few other customers were present. Guided by teachers and teacher aides, the children chattered with excitement. Difficult decisions were made more difficult by eyes unable to see the 33-flavor listings. In their joy, the children pressed against the counter windows, anxious to taste the ice cream. All except Everett!

He, too, had first started to think of serving himself. Then he remembered their guest. Quickly he made his way to Mr. Williamson. He pushed the wheelchair up to a table and then waited on Ralph.

When they arrived back at the school, Mrs. Summers used this event to illustrate a lesson. For these kids and ourselves the example of serving others before serving ourselves needs to be pointed out.

When Everett was nine, our friends Lee and Kathy Dimmick were planning a move to a new house. Most people would decline to baby-sit under those circumstances. They knew, however, that Mary Lee and I were hoping to attend a Christian convention in Denver, Colorado. We had been unable to attend such events since Everett Lee was born, but his health now permitted us to consider it. With Everett's history of crisis illnesses, though, even close friends and relatives were still reluctant to care for him.

The Dimmicks, however, were the exception. They assured us, "He won't be an inconvenience. We'll just put him to work helping us move."

So we took the trip, assured that our kids were well cared for. After 2500 miles, we returned home, refreshed in body, soul, and spirit.

At the Dimmicks' Everett Lee announced, "I helped!" We learned that our son had indeed helped. With Lee's patient coaching and management, Everett had done what he could with his awkward hands and legs. Carefully cradling an object in the crook of the "lazy" right arm and holding it with the stronger left hand, he had made trip after trip. From the truck to the house he had carried one item at a time and then returned for another. Lee told me, "He never said 'I can't!' " We were grateful for their patience in letting him participate.

God used many people to impart the attitude of which Lee spoke. Good friends, wonderful teachers, and his family all tried to support Everett's "I can" spirit. However, a verse we memorized together was the real key: "I can do all things through Him who strengthens me" (Phil. 4:13).

Everett was very quick to point to the Source. The first half of the verse would have made no sense at all without the power named in the second half. We talked freely with him about the ways in which God works in our lives each day. He capably interpreted the events of his life as well as or better than we. All of us knew that for this boy every "I can" was a gift from God.

When there was a chance to share in our church services, Everett was always ready with a song selection or a meaningful prayer request. Sometimes I would ask the congregation to tell recent examples of God's goodness to them. Everett Lee's physical vision was poor, but his contributions indicated unusually well-developed spiritual vision. On other evenings we would quote favorite verses. Immediately his hand would shoot up. It was always first! On occasion I would urge him to let others have a chance to speak by moving on to someone else. But this boy was always ready to give an answer to anyone who asked about the hope that was within him (1 Peter 3:15).

In most cases his quick response gave inspiration, but sometimes it brought smiles. At an area-wide church rally, the program had been completed. Just before the benediction prayer, I called for the churches represented to identify themselves. When each of them was named, the delegation stood for recognition. I concluded by asking, "Have I missed anyone?"

Everett Lee popped up and said, "Daddy, you forgot our church!"

Indeed! His unique way of pointing out my error brought a wave of chuckles. The oversight was remedied and the closing prayer given. I had hardly opened my eyes when he was at my side by the front pew. He proudly asked, "Aren't you glad I told you about forgetting us?"

"I sure am, young man."

He was excited to be of any service in the life of the church. He did everything he possibly could, in living rebuke of those who won't attempt things because they "can't."

Junior choir was the first real opportunity open to Everett. Here he could combine his love of song and love of witness. The director was nearly run over by his enthusiasm. She often had to caution him to blend in with the others. Otherwise, she would have had a one-voice choir accompanied by 18 children pantomiming. He adapted to her instruction and became valuable to the choir.

One of his proudest moments came when Angie Bartel asked him, "Everett, will you lead songs for junior church next month?"

His prompt reply was, "I'll be glad to do it."

In the next weeks he gave much thought to each song. Many of the selections were his favorites. The communion hymn was picked with the greatest possible care. He took the responsibility very seriously, and he did an excellent job.

The boy whose eyes could scarcely read the titles and whose hands struggled to hold the book made a good leader. He led us all to see the joy of doing what we can. God doesn't ask us to do more than that. In Everett Lee we discovered that most of us miss many of God's intended blessings by doing less than we can.

He was bold to tell people of God's goodness to him. Another verse our family committed to memory was Romans 1:16: "For I am not ashamed of the gospel, for it is the power of God for salvation to everyone who believes, to the Jew first and also to the Greek."

Everett Lee loved to ride with Ken Jensen on the Sunday school bus route, and Ken, in turn, was pleased to have him on board. His warm spirit and positive enthusiasm added to the welcome extended to the early morning riders. Everett was a fixture in the seat right behind the driver.

Ken related an incident from one of their morning drives. As they were traveling down a residential street, Everett Lee spotted a young boy playing in a driveway. He insisted that Ken stop the bus so that he could invite the boy to Sunday school. Ken complied.

With his usual difficulty, Everett climbed down the steep steps and carefully crossed the street. A friendly word of greeting and an invitation was extended to the other lad. As he climbed back aboard, Everett reported that the boy was interested in attending church services. They pulled away from the curb, with the boy in the yard and the boy on the bus waving to each other.

"Father, thank you for the example of love and service you have given us in our son. Please help us grow more sensitive to the hurts and needs of those around us, and may the beauty of Jesus be seen in me as clearly as it was in Everett Lee."

CHAPTER THIRTEEN

Believable Faith

"Do you know what that cross up there makes me think about?"

This question came from Everett Lee as we sat down to dinner. The day before, a cross had been added to the gabled bell tower of the church building on Skyline Road. Fifteen years earlier the designers had planned for a steeple to be located on the tower, but other priorities had been placed ahead of that project. Now the view from our dining room revealed a graceful white cross overshadowing the long roof line of the church.

"No, Everett. What does the new steeple make you think about?"

"It makes me think about 'Jesus, Keep Me Near the Cross.'"

Inwardly we rejoiced that Everett was able to

see the new spire at all. Moreover, the example of his spiritual growth challenged us.

For nine years this boy prompted spiritual growth in those around him. Originally this growth was born out of the immense problems at his birth. Mom and Dad, brother and sisters had been forced to dig deeper into God's Word. It is easy to profess faith when all is well, but the hard times of testing are the means by which our faith deepens. During our "testing times," the Lord calls us to test him. He wants to show himself faithful. In many times of insufficiency we tried God and found him sufficient.

As Everett Lee gained ability to reason and understand, he always seemed to see God's power and God's Word as the center of his life. My wife's faith is simple and complete, and she diligently shared it with him, praying that God would use her. Bible-story reading and a steady flow of gospel music showed Jesus to our family. Dinner time and bedtime were special guidance periods. The young woman I had married taught daily in that important classroom, our home.

Everett's faith seemed without a beginning. It just blossomed and grew. Perhaps in being less distracted by visual things, he was free to excel as a student in the class on faith. In 2 Corinthians 5:7 we learn that our walk is to be "by faith, not by sight."

He seemed to understand the faith-walk better than we do who have no visual handicap. Many of us say, "I'll believe it when I see it." Everett simply believed, and then God showed him what many will never see because they lack faith.

When Everett was five I returned from a seminar in Wheaton, Illinois, with a new tool for spiritually equipping our family. We began keeping "life notebooks." We all acquired three-ring binders reflecting something of our different personalities. Everett's, of course, had a bright green cover. Each week for many months we spent Sunday afternoons happily cutting out pictures to illustrate spiritual truths. We sang favorite songs and recited verses, with rewards given for accurately quoting scripture.

The opening sections of our notebooks were devoted to the spiritual meanings of our names. In the seminar it was pointed out that all the names from the Old and New Testament eras have meaning. God directed that the meanings symbolize positive spiritual achievement for those in his family. Names were changed when the meaning became inappropriate due to a major change in a life. Abram to Abraham, Sarai to Sarah, Jacob to Israel, and Simon to Peter are but a few examples.

We experienced real joy as we researched the cultural definitions of our names and attached the spiritual meanings to them. This section in our life notebooks became the focus of many exciting discoveries in our Bible reading. We recorded the verses of scripture that became personal challenges from the Lord to us.

We were startled to learn that the traits in the spiritual meaning of our kids' names were "custom fit." Frederick, our rugged and attractive oldest son, was to be a "peaceful ruler." Quiet and sensitive Jo Ann is indeed a picture of "God's grace." Frisky and freckled Kathy was called to be "God's pure one." Everett, with his special history, was found to be "strong and brave." The life verses stemming from these meanings continue to inspire us.

Mary Lee and I were concerned that the goals envisioned by the meaning of the children's names be sought in the power of God, so one of the first verses we learned around the family circle was: "Trust in the Lord with all your heart, and do not lean on your own understanding. In all your ways acknowledge Him, and He will make your paths straight" (Prov. 3:5-6).

Soon we also learned 1 Corinthians 3:11: "For no man can lay a foundation other than the one which is laid, which is Jesus Christ."

Everett Lee learned the verses flawlessly and the lessons very well. He trusted the Lord completely for his bravery and strength. He rested his life firmly upon Jesus, the sure foundation. When he stood and quoted these verses, listeners knew he understood and believed what was said.

A family vacation in Eastern Oregon provided insights which we added for permanent reference to the pages of our life notebooks. Everett Lee had just turned seven when we went on a week-long camping trip. The vacation, which included Grandma and Grandpa Payton, is one of our best memories. We camped practically alone on the Grande

Rhonde River near LaGrand, Oregon. This country, for which the Nez Pierce Indians and Chief Joseph fought so hard, is an inspiration. The high meadows are surrounded by rugged mountains. Pine and tamarack and fir trees ascend from the lush green meadows to snowcapped peaks. The river below our camp began as creeks winding through those meadows. The streams converged to rush through a gash in the stone cliffs.

We all hiked to a hillside opening in the forest, where we settled down in the tall grass under the massive single pine tree in the center of the clearing. My parents had recently received a recording of the funeral memorial service for a distant relative. Warren McIntire had served the Lord with great zest and commitment until his death at 91. With the sun shining down on us, we listened to the tribute paid to a life of great faith and service. At times we stopped the tape while the grandparents shared additions from their own treasury of faith. We all were deeply inspired by the commentary on this man's life.

We came down from that mountain having gained more esteem for the victorious Christian life. Everett Lee was very attentive. With his hand in Grandma's, he was unusually thoughtful for a seven-year-old. The two of them reminded me of Paul's observation about the faith of young Timothy: "For I am mindful of the sincere faith within you, which first dwelt in your grandmother Lois, and your mother Eunice" (2 Tim. 1:5).

Everett had heard a message of truth from those

he loved and trusted utterly. Through the lips and life of Mother and Grandmother, reinforced by Dad and Granddad, the truth had been spoken. Everett had listened carefully and embraced the testimony in word and song that afternoon: "Only one life will soon be past. Only what's done for Christ will last."

Our family gathers in another moment of drama each Sunday morning. Before going to Sunday school, we assemble around the dining table. To make the meaning and blessing of our offering gifts a family experience, we have secured stewardship envelopes for each of our children. To avoid training them in penny ante giving, we divide the tithe of our total family income among the givers. Mom and Dad have the largest portions, which the youngsters understand.

Everett nearly always led the way to the table in this preparation for worship. "Come on, you guys, it's time to pray for our offerings," he urged, adding, "I'll get the offering envelopes."

Dad passed several dollar bills to each one in the circle and circulated a pen for writing the amount on the envelopes. Everett struggled to write the number himself. A time of prayer followed. We wanted to tell the Lord we really knew that everything we have is from him. Everett Lee was always ready to express our cheerfulness in dedicating these dollars back to God. In stewardship faith, as in other areas, Everett led the way for the others around that table. He embodied the words of the prophet: "A little boy will lead them" (Isa. 11:6).

"Father, thank you for the knowledge and trust of the Savior given to Everett Lee. And thank you for the way he has caused our faith to grow. You have shown your goodness to us through his glowing testimony."

Everett Lee's complete trust and love for the Word of God sparkled brilliantly. Many saw and were challenged by his eagerness to study the large-print edition of the Scriptures which God permitted him to read. He memorized numerous verses which were indeed a lamp to his feet and a light to his path (Ps. 119:105). By God's Word he could see!

Kathy Moskal, a high school neighbor girl, received the following classroom assignment several months after Everett Lee's death: "Name the person, other than your parents, who has most affected your life." She wrote:

> Everett Lee Payton is the only person that really influenced my life besides my parents. He was always happy. With all his problems, he still trusted Christ and knew almost every verse you asked him. That's the way he influenced me. He made me want to be a better Christian. When he died, I took his life verse as my own . . . "I will be brave and strong, banishing all fear and doubt, For the Lord my God is with me wherever I go" (Josh. 1:9).

CHAPTER FOURTEEN

Impossible Dreams?

God is so good. (Hallelujah!)
God is so good. (Hallelujah!)
God is so good, He's so good to me.

Our family often sang this chorus at church and at home. Everett Lee always inserted the "Hallelujah!" He heard a group of teens who had returned from camp sing it that way. Forever after, this was his personal signature, endorsing the truth of which we sang. The Hebrew word "hallelujah" means "praise the Lord." We could only nod our agreement when he soloed on this addition to the chorus.

God had certainly been very good to Everett. Mary Lee and I knew that God had indeed been good to us, also. Our prayers were being answered. Everett's progress had exceeded any medical expectations. He was handicapped in obvious ways, and crisis moments had been plentiful, but the deepest longings of our hearts were being fulfilled by a generous and loving God. Our cry to God for impossible things was heard. In our weakness and in Everett's, the Lord was showing himself strong.

We had asked specifically for three things. First we asked that Everett Lee have a good mind. The tiny "not big enough for real intelligence" brain had been blessed by the hands of Jesus like the loaves and fishes beside Galilee. The second and third cries from our hearts, those longings which God was honoring most of all, were for Everett to come to know the Lord and to bring glory to the Savior.

Grandma Rosin, an 88-year-old saint, reminded us that others were with us in prayer. In her heavy German accent, she asked one day about Everett Lee's health and progress. Then she said, "I pray for that boy every day, you know."

We were at once humbled. God was answering our prayers. But we knew that the prayers of this dear woman and others like her were keys to the results. Noting all these blessings, we prayed, "Father, thank you for granting the impossible to Everett. Thank you for fulfilling our longings for him. May the life of our broken doll continue to bring praise to you."

Everett Lee's own words of praise directed the attention of those who knew him to God's goodness. The words of Jesus were true: "Out of the mouth of babes and sucklings thou hast perfected praise" (Matt. 21:16 KJV).

Everett's words were simple, yet eloquent. He

often said, "God has been so good to me." His hallelujahs punctuated the testimony.

We recognize honestly that Everett Lee was never a "normal" boy. He was gifted with miracle vision, but those eyes never saw with normal efficiency. The simplest activities required unusual concentration and terrific effort. One leg always dragged, and one of his arms never functioned properly. He was always dependent on the hidden shunt pump in his skull. Still, he was able to experience normal things. And, in a special way, the abnormalities turned a floodlight on the power and presence of God.

Everett's favorite game, Trouble, was a parable of the life he was living. In this table game, a pair of dice are housed beneath a clear plastic dome in the center of the playing board. The dome is pressed and released to shake the dice. The players move colored pegs around the board, attempting to get them into home base. Opposing players bump others' pegs back to the start by landing on their spaces.

Everett strained to see the number of dots on the dice. Others "popped" the dice with ease, but for him it was hard work. Yet, win or lose, his enthusiasm for Trouble was ever present. There was an aura of victory in his approach to this frustrating game, quite like his approach to problems in real life. Trouble was something he had learned to live with.

Most children collect one thing or another—rocks or coins or stamps. Everett had a collection too. Coin banks lined his shelves. Because he showed much joy when he received the first couple of banks, they just kept coming. On birthdays or at Christmas, one of his many friends would remember the piggy-bank collection. It came to be a source of personal pride.

Everett's banks did not represent the stashing of coins. Money was never important to him, except on Sunday mornings. But showing appreciation when a bank was given was important to him. And the pleasure others expressed when he invited them to see his banks was important, too.

The Payton family does engage in one coin-saving project each year. We attempt to finance our family vacations by saving quarters. Everett Lee was a happy participant in this project. With the other three youngsters, he helped count the dwindling treasury at the end of each travel day, making neat little stacks of the remaining quarters. Then we discussed what we could do for the balance of our vacation, weighing wishes against the number of coins and voting on the suggestions.

One annual suggestion was a surefire winner: Fred and Daddy playing a round of golf. The spectators would accompany the participants in a rented golf cart. Everett Lee loved to "help drive." Also, he was pleased to assist in tending the flag when we reached the greens. "Which way on this hole?" he would ask. We would point the direction down the next fairway. He could scarcely see beyond the women's tee box, but, accepting the matter by faith, he would say, "Hit a big one, Daddy!"

Most of our family vacations were on the Oregon coast. We enjoyed many fascinating commercial activities in this area, but we preferred exploring natural beauty. A family hike through forests or wind-swept dunes is unexcelled for inspiration and refreshment. Our activities were often strenuous, but Everett Lee walked every foot of these hikes with us. Few youngsters have covered more territory. His brother or sisters helped by lifting him over obstacles.

Watching them, I was reminded of an account of a young boy who daily was seen carrying a still younger family member around the neighborhood. The smaller lad's legs were twisted and useless. A bystander asked the older boy, "Isn't the little fellow an awful burden to you?" To which he replied, "Mister, he's no burden. He's my brother."

Our kids were helping Everett Lee do all the normal things. Sharing in these activities had been part of our longings for him. All of us felt glad for every moment and every place we could enjoy together. Any effort was worth it, and Everett was not considered a burden.

One summer we accepted the challenge of scaling the steep south side of Cape Kiawanda. The cape extends half a mile into the surging ocean. At points it is 100 or more feet high. From the top the view of the awesome Pacific is breathtaking.

Our climb was to be up the sheer face of dry sand. We began on the beach, with the vegetation on the top our goal. The six of us were accompanied by Duchess, a recent addition to our family.

The big Saint Bernard positioned herself at Everett Lee's side, taking charge of his needs. She caught him as the sand began to slide. Then, with her shoulders, she pushed him upward.

Progress was very slow for the whole group. We were taking one step forward and sliding back two. We took long pauses to regain the strength in our quivering legs and to catch our breath. But when we reached the top, we drank deeply of the sky, land, and sea shimmering before us. Basking in the sun and breeze, we laughed about Everett Lee's guide dog.

A few months earlier, our family had attended a charity auction. One of the first items placed on sale was a 10-month-old Saint Bernard. Our kids begged me to bid, but I remained silent. I realized the dog was worth at least $100. More pleading followed. Mary Lee and I were sure the sad-eyed animal would sell for a good deal of money, so to appease the kids we let Fred bid $10. To our dismay, there were no other bids! In a state of shock, we took hold of the leash and started for the car.

This crazy accident turned out to be a blessing. Everett was fearful of most dogs, with their quick moves, but he loved this one. She moved more slowly and was big enough for him to touch easily. And we were pleasantly surprised that, in spite of her size, she was less costly to keep than dogs we had previously owned.

Do you think God cares about things like a special boy having a special dog? Even by this auction "mistake," God was being good to our son.

In many ways the Lord was fulfilling our desire for Everett Lee to live as normally as possible. In fact, Everett came to have more than ordinary opportunities. Through the efforts of loved ones in and out of our family, he camped out, rode in a private airplane, rode a train, rode an elephant, and rode his brother's horse. He met and talked to James Irwin, astronaut; Norma Zimmer, singer; Paul Harvey, newscaster; Stuart Hamblen, song writer; and McCall and Straub, governors of Oregon.

Indeed, God was filling our son's life. Already two of Everett Lee's greatest longings had been granted: He had been baptized into Jesus Christ, and people liked him. His other two longings were yet to be fulfilled. The first was the desire to attend his "own week" of Christian Service Camp. The other was to be reunited with his Grandma Hayes, who had died when he was six years old. A number of times he said, "I can't wait to see Grandma." Both of these remaining wishes would be granted in his climactic ninth year.

The words of another song by Bill Gaither expressed Everett Lee's feelings very well. In a morning hour of worship, he sang:

I Guess God Thought of Everything

I'm glad God gave me arms
to hold my daddy tight,
And legs to run and meet him
when he comes home at night;

And I can feel the warmth
of the fireplace at night,
    I guess God thought of Everything.

My eyes can see the diamonds
when moonlight's on the snow,
My ears can hear the birds sing,
the friendly rooster crow;
My nose can smell warm spices
of cookies in a row,
    I guess God thought of Everything.

God knew I'd need a family
to make a house a home,
He knew I'd need a place
where I could be alone;
And clothes to fit my body,
a warm bed of my own,
    I guess God thought of Everything.

CHAPTER FIFTEEN

Nine Already

THE EXCITEMENT and beauty of the Rose Festival had heralded Everett Lee's birth. Now, as we anticipated his ninth birthday, a far larger celebration was approaching. The United States of America was nearing its 200th anniversary.

"*Old 4449* is coming!"

"What's *Old 4449?*" the kids asked.

I explained: "It's a huge, steam-powered locomotive. The early trains in our country were all pulled by steam engines until modern diesel engines replaced them years ago. This big locomotive was resting and rusting in Portland. Now *Old 4449* has been restored and made like new. It will pull the *Freedom Train*, filled with some of America's great historical documents, across all of America."

This vehicle out of the past had caught my imagination, and I wanted it to catch the imagination of my children. The steel and smoke and collection of memorabilia were less important than the history and enthusiasm for America they symbolized. I wanted to put my kids in touch with the past and instill in them a sense of patriotism.

For the next several days we tantalized each other with the prospect of the train's arrival.

"You won't believe those eight-foot-six-inch wheels churning down the tracks!"

"Yeah, and the paper says the whistle is something else."

The *Freedom Train* was to pull into Salem on the first leg of its nationwide journey at 2:45 A.M. Saturday. We wanted to see it arriving. Anything for which a family sets their alarm clocks for 2:00 A.M. is memorable. This was to be a "happening."

Five of us arose quickly at the sound of the alarm. Everett Lee had to be reminded briefly of how "neat" this experience was going to be. Then he too shook off the cobwebs of sleep.

We drove through the deserted downtown streets to the planned spot. The Southern Pacific rail line splits Salem in two at the middle. In a darkened service station lot, we took position. Facing across Twelfth Street, we could see the glistening ribbon of steel for a quarter of a mile in both directions. The time was 2:30 A.M.

A few other hardy souls were seen waiting at similar posts. We waited . . . and waited . . . and waited some more! Problems of switching tracks up the line delayed the arrival of the immense engine. Three or four of us slept in shifts as the others watched. We started the cold car a couple of times and drove around the block. After almost three and a half hours, we all agreed to drive to a donut shop. Just as we saw the sign outside of the shop, a shrill shriek pierced the air.

"That's it! That's the steam whistle!" I yelled.

We whirled the car around and back. The brilliant headlight of *Old 4449*, towering above her cowcatcher, met our headlights as we turned onto Twelfth Street again. She was moving slowly. A number of cars joined us in the half-mile drive paralleling the track. We moved at five miles per hour, hypnotized by those huge wheels directly across the empty lane of opposing traffic.

All the kids' faces were jammed against the windows. The long wait had been worth it! This vantage point was better than we had hoped for. Instead of watching the train go by, we escorted her to the place of her three-day display.

Everett Lee asked, "What's all that white stuff?"

"That's the steam!" we answered in a chorus.

Wrapped in the cloud of vapor trailing the engine, the rest of the train had a ghostlike quality. That ancient piece of machinery painted red, white, and blue was a thing of beauty. It seemed alive with personality.

In the dim light of dawn, we walked the length of the train. That afternoon we returned to inspect its interior. The *Freedom Train* intensified the Paytons' love for our country and our heritage under God. Those rolling wheels carried the bicentennial celebration into our town. They also ushered in Everett Lee's climactic year.

One of the big events for Everett that year was a special week of camp. The National Camps for the Blind invited him to a week at Sunset Lake. Mary Lee and I trembled a little at the thought of his traveling as far as Tacoma, Washington, but after much prayer we filled out the forms. A camp representative assured us that top-quality medical personnel would be present. We sent Everett's medical history to the camp nurse.

The Salem kids attending the camp would be leaving by bus at 8:00 A.M. We intended to eat breakfast together at a nearby restaurant, but we were delayed. We arrived at the restaurant with only 20 minutes to spare. Four of us decided to order coffee or milk and a breakfast roll to go. While Jo Ann stayed with Everett Lee to have a more substantial breakfast, we drove to the waiting bus to load his gear and make sure they didn't pull away without him.

The suitcases and sleeping bags had all been placed in the rear of the bus. All but two of the youngsters were already aboard and waiting to begin the trip. Soon Everett Lee and Jo Ann appeared. As they walked toward us, hand in hand, we noticed the stony silence on the bus. The two drivers were outside making a last check on the vehicle. The kids were spaced widely on the big bus. None were smiling, and all were absolutely still. When Jo and Everett drew close, we stepped toward them to hug and kiss him good-bye. Then we assisted him up the steep steps.

With a wide smile, he climbed on board. The others were listening to determine who the new passenger was. Making another step into the aisle, as if knowing they needed a clue, he announced himself: "Hi, sweethearts!"

The soundless group broke into excited chatter. Every face wore a smile as they greeted the new arrival. They sounded like a cageful of magpies. There would be a few more minutes of waiting, but the fun of the trip had already begun. It had started with the greeting of a crippled boy who had pulled himself up to join his sightless friends.

These handicapped youngsters had a great week. They came home with tales of horseback riding, swimming, and archery. Everett Lee enjoyed the distinction of having been thrown into the lake with his clothes on, but he was not a clown all of the time. We learned that once again he had served as chaplain.

After his ninth birthday, Everett exclaimed several times, "Mommy, can you believe I'm nine already?"

Or he would ask, "Daddy, can you believe you've had me for nine whole years?"

Looking at each other with spirits united in love, we replied, "No, Everett. We can't believe we've had you for nine years already. God surely has been good to us."

"Father, thank you for the difference those nine years made in all of our lives."

CHAPTER SIXTEEN

Camper of the Week

"MOMMY, what if someone makes fun of me at camp?"

This unexpected question came several months before Everett's long anticipated "week of my very own" at fourth-fifth-sixth-grade camp. This trip would fulfill years of longings, and he was already living it in his mind.

A firm wall of protective love had followed him everywhere. The environment at school, at church, and at home constantly took into account his limitations. Now real alarm crept in. Among 140 children, he could be the only one with handicaps of sight and motion. The question was an aftershock of facing this truth.

"I don't know, Everett. What do you think you'll do if someone makes fun of you?" He'd caught Mary Lee off-guard.

He replied soberly, "Maybe I'll cry a little." But then quickly, as if correcting a grave mistake, "No, I won't cry. My name is Everett. I am strong and brave."

The little wedge of fear, which might have produced a major change in his personality, had been banished. God's word in Joshua 1:9 had issued forth to wash away the hazard to his uncrippled spirit.

It was very easy for Everett to live in advance the coming days in August. Wi-Ne-Ma Christian Camp had been a regular retreat sight for our family during all of his years. We had spent at least one week each summer in our tent under the twisted coastal pines.

In the tribal tongue "Wi-Ne-Ma" means "Beautiful Lady of the Lake." Everett Lee and she had fallen in love some time ago. Fred, Jo Ann, and Kathy related stories of their camping experiences, increasing Everett's infatuation. Finally the dreams so real for several years were to come true. He was to attend his very own week of camp.

The trip from Salem to Wi-Ne-Ma usually takes 90 minutes. On some occasions, however, it seems much longer because of the strong desire to arrive. The kids were especially eager on this trip.

Generally the first item of business at camp is registration, when assignments are made to sleeping quarters. Then counselors escort the kids to their cabins, helping with their gear.

Everett Lee, though, was thinking of a higher priority. The car doors had scarcely closed behind them when he stood before a special friend and asked, "Will you go to the banquet with me, Nancy?"

The campers call the Friday-night meal "the banquet." The cooks, who do an outstanding job all week, really give Friday night something extra. The kids decorate the dining hall and tables. In junior-level camps, there is no suggestion of dates for that evening, but there is some dating in upper-grade camps, and Everett Lee had heard the big boys tell all about it.

Pretty little Nancy Woodruff was very special to him. She treated him with kindness and warmth. They had a wonderful relationship. Both were far from understanding the complexities of big kids' dating, but, by close association in the church family, a healthy and lovely mutual admiration had developed between them.

Everett wanted her commitment to share the camp banquet highlight. She gave it willingly. With this important task satisfactorily completed, he could give attention to other activities.

This camp is structured around the Word of God. Several classes are offered in the mornings. A missions chapel precedes lunch and features a missionary guest. Ample recreation fills the afternoon, with such supervised options as swimming in the ocean or lake, boating, and playing in the dunes. Evenings provide time for crafts, dramas, and talent shows. The bonfire song and inspiration service by the lake conclude each full day, and the counselors have no trouble getting their troops to sleep.

By then, all energies are spent, and pillows never looked better.

Everett entered into each facet of camp with every ounce of his ability. He devoured the class instruction. He sat in the front row in chapel. Those uncooperative legs carried him to the lake for swimming every day, and often to the top of the slide.

The Giant Sky Slide had been purchased by Wi-Ne-Ma for $1200 when an amusement park declared bankruptcy. The original cost of the 30-feet-tall, fiber-glass slide and its steel framework was $20,000. Those of us who watched Everett Lee and scores of others climb the 44 steps and descend, screaming with joy, rejoiced at how God provides good things and fun times for those who love him.

Despite the fun, however, Everett was feeling the pain of a situation not constructed with a handicapped child in mind. The staff and kids were kind, but he was sometimes frustrated. Our Kathy, who was among the sixth graders there, worked hard at being far away, yet close at hand for this boy so near to her heart.

Everett broke down once two days into the week. Privately he cried to her, "Kathy, I don't have any friends!"

She helped him over this hurdle. The statement was the furthest thing from the truth. But perhaps for the first time in his life, Everett was hurting from being left a little behind. This feeling was as visible on the hike to the picnic as it had been in the tearful statement to Kathy.

For one lunch each week, the cooks plan a picnic on the beach. A large rock formation about a mile and a half up the beach forms two walls of the outside dining room. The surf, with shells and agates at its edge, fascinates the kids.

Soft sand makes a tiring walk for all, and appetites are increased for the customary hot dogs and potato salad. Glen Lyda, camp manager and long-time close friend of our family, takes all the food to the meal site on a tractor. One or two faculty members often ride with him to and from the picnic. That day Glen sought Everett Lee and invited him to ride. Usually the offer to mount the tractor would have brought an excited "Yes!" But not this time. "Thank you, Glen," he said. "I'd rather walk with all the other guys."

And he did. With great effort he kept up with all the rest. It may be that he had something to prove to himself. He certainly showed everyone else his determination.

Eldon Barnes, boys' dean for the week, was one of the first to welcome Everett on the opening day of camp. From that moment on, this kind man watched over many of our son's needs. He gave much assistance in tying shoes, grooming, and reminding of medication times. Also, he was very sensitive about any youngsters making fun of Everett Lee.

Glen related later that, one afternoon as he and Eldon were talking, Eldon's face suddenly flushed with color. With a quick wave, he excused himself. The dean, a man of near 60, ran off down the dirt road that passes through the camp. In a few minutes he came walking back, somewhat winded.

"I thought a boy down there was mimicking Everett Lee." With a sheepish grin, he reported, "I got clear down there and found out it was Everett Lee himself!" The two men shook with laughter at this false alarm.

For many people the talent show was the most memorable evening of the week. Everett Lee had gone to camp with a song in mind that he wanted to sing during chapel or at some other appropriate time. When talent night arrived, he had not sung it yet, so Kathy urged him to do it in the show. He agreed, but was too late to be included in the program of the competing groups. Hence, the program director simply added it to the end of the schedule.

Toward the close of the hour, after a number of fine selections had been shared by gifted young people, Everett was called upon. He stepped up onto the little platform. With shoulders back and head up, he sang this song by Bill and Gloria Gaither.

I Am a Promise

I am a promise, I am a possibility,
I am a promise—with a capital "P."
I am a great big bundle of potentiality.
And I am learnin'—to hear God's voice,
And I am tryin' to make the right choice,

I'm a promise to be—
    anything God wants me to be.

I can go anywhere He wants me to go,
I can be anything that He wants me to be,
I can climb the high mountains,
I can cross the wide sea,
I'm a great big promise, you see!

I am a promise, I am a possibility,
I am a promise—with a capital "P."
I am a great big bundle of potentiality
And I am learnin'—to hear God's voice,
And I am tryin' to make the right choice,
I'm a promise to be—
    anything God wants me to be.

As he finished this testimony, every person in the building rose to his feet. Deafening applause continued for several minutes. Many of the faculty and youngsters clapped while tears streamed down their faces.

God had done it again. Dramatically, he had used Everett Lee to bring glory to the Lord Jesus Christ. In a way uniquely his, Everett directed all of the applause heavenward.

Don Spencer was the young director of this camp week. When he learned of our son's death, he wrote, "The picture is engraved upon my soul. Everett stood tall, struggling a bit to get those words out. . . . This image will be a lifelong inspiration to me. I praise God for that one week of life with Everett Lee."

The guest missionary for this week was Madonna Burget. Her ministry is with children in India. A registered nurse, she was able to double as missions speaker and nurse at the camp. She later wrote in *Jet Cadet* magazine:

> The week at Wi-Ne-Ma was unforgettable to me, mostly because of Everett Lee. He came to me in the morning and evening for medications. There was seldom a time that he didn't say, "I love you, Madonna. You are my favorite nurse. Will you come back next year and be my nurse?"

She told him she could not come back next year. In a few months she planned to be in India once more. She concluded:

> He will not be back at Wi-Ne-Ma next year either. Everett will be with his Lord in heaven. I can see him now looking up at Jesus and saying, "I love you, Jesus!" Yes, Everett Lee was a promise. He was also a blessing to all who crossed his path. I will be unable to remember all the children that I met in that week. But I will never forget Everett.

This dedicated woman knew much about the nature of Everett's hydrocephalus and cerebral palsy, yet she recognized this boy as a Promise with a capital P. For her and all the others present, Everett's problems only magnified the witness of his life to the power of God.

"Father, thank you for fulfilling Everett Lee's longings. Thank you for giving him Joshua 1:9 and Philippians 4:13. And thank you, Father, for all the wonderful promises that are ours through the Lord Jesus Christ."

CHAPTER SEVENTEEN

The Family Hunt

A SLOGAN that has stood the test of time is "The family that prays together stays together." Through these years we have found this call to spiritual union meaningful and true. The heart and core of our family life is bound together by the presence of God.

With prayer at the center, a new turn of the old slogan has come to be important to us. "The family that *plays* together stays together" are words of wisdom at our house. I commend them to you as good mortar in building on the foundation of Jesus Christ.

For several years it appeared that Mary Lee and I were making an exception to family unity by going elk hunting and leaving our children at home. Eventually, however, the family hunting trip would become the final and finest expression of our togetherness.

Hunting was new for Mary Lee and me. Neither of us was raised in a family that hunted. In fact, no one in either family had ever owned a rifle. However, we have always loved the out-of-doors. From our first exposure to the sport, we were infected by the vigor and challenge of elk hunting. We could hardly wait to share the joy of this strenuous camping experience with our kids.

Roy and Alta Beckwith fanned that initial spark of enthusiasm in us. Roy, an elder in our church, is a man I respect very much. The early-November trip is a family affair to the Beckwiths, so they were able to disarm any negative feelings we had had about hunting. We could see our four joining this expedition when they grew older.

In the meantime, for each of our children the hunting trip meant a short visit at Grandma's or their cousins' house. Everett Lee's health was improved, but during these days he stayed with the relatives nearest to the doctor and hospital facilities. While the children gladly shared in our anticipation of and planning for the trip, we still all eagerly awaited the year when it would be possible for us to go hunting together.

Until then, tales of tenting with a wood stove in zero to 25 degree temperatures, and oftentimes snow, would have to satisfy. We painted pictures in their minds of the mountains and meadows with ice-cold streams. Their imaginations were gripped by reported sightings of big game animals and by occasional success in the hunt.

As we prepared to leave, Everett would say, "I hope you catch one, Daddy!"

But as we pulled away on the start of the 300-mile trip, the kids knew our objective was recreation. The car and the little trailer were loaded with expectations of fun and fellowship, in addition to equipment. Our children knew that success in this change-of-pace trip would be measured in terms of vigorous refreshment.

Twice we spent some wonderful summer days camping with our kids in the hunting area. Warmed by the summer sun, we walked the game trails and ridges under the towering Anthony Buttes. One Sunday morning we rose at 3:30 to climb a mountain called Bobcat. With a fantastic view of the surrounding mountains and valleys, we watched the sun come up. We sang and worshiped God, who we knew had created it all. Then, circling a small bonfire, we shared in the Communion Christ instituted by saying, "Do this in remembrance of me."

While facing the sunrise, we had not noticed the dark clouds moving in from the west. Descending the mountain, our children glimpsed the sudden fury of a high-mountain storm. Thunder and lightning put on a Sunday-morning show, followed by torrential rain falling on our tent. The fascinations of the place Mom and Dad had talked about had become real to our children.

That fall Everett was nine. I had a strong sense

of urgency that this should be the year of our family hunt, although our busy schedule seemed, at first, to prohibit this plan. Fred was playing starting tackle on the football team. A new field of work was just beginning for Mary Lee. And my responsibilities seemed especially pressing. But my impression was nevertheless very strong. If all of us were to enjoy a hunting trip together, it had to be this year.

Preparations for this excursion were more elaborate than for any other. Complicating circumstances were plentiful, including a very limited budget. However, as Halloween neared, our household reached a high pitch of excitement. We were elated by astonishing solutions to many of the complex problems that could have prevented us from making the trip. At last we all would be enjoying this outing together.

The trip began on a Thursday evening. By driving all night, we would reach the isolated campsite early the day before hunting season was to open. Then we would have Friday to set up tents, stoves, tarps, and beds.

A continuous line of taillights stretched before us. This annual trek of trucks and trailers reminds us of the covered wagon trains moving westward on the same route many years ago. Those in this modern wagon train show similar planning and commitment to meet the challenges of the rugged land.

Roy and Alta had arrived with Charles Crane at the selected campsite on the day before. The

Dimmicks and our family completed the hunting community of several years' standing. Part of this special season were Steve and Diane Turner and their three children. Roy had hung a red towel from a pole to mark the spot for us to pull off the logging road. We could scarcely see their trailer at our destination in the clearing 50 yards away. Tents and trailers formed a little circle in the clearing, hardly disturbing the serenity of the wilderness.

Once we were there, everyone helped to set up our camp. A hundred jobs had to be done before we could relax for the evening meal by lantern light. Everett Lee chipped in, unpacking and carrying wood.

A few weeks before, Everett Lee had been "caught" in Daddy's bed. In the exchange that followed, I announced I would throw him in a snowbank when we went hunting. In the intervening weeks, he reminded me, "You're not really going to throw me in the snow, are you, Daddy?" When I confirmed my intention, he would giggle and say, "Oh boy. Oh boy."

But there was no snow around our camping area on this trip. In fact, this was an unusually fine season of bluebird weather. The heavy clothing required in the severe cold of the mornings was shed before noon on very mild and sunny days. The good weather was a blessing, with so many young ones on the outing.

All of us got a look at some elk. None were bulls, so they did not end up gracing our table, but what excitement! It is a thrill just to glimpse these big, agile animals. Some hunters nurture for several years the memory of one close viewing.

One afternoon Alta Beckwith was leading the women and children on a hike. Standing among the trees that bordered an open slash area, they heard snapping twigs. Five elk stepped into the opening. The wind was right so the animals detected no scent, and they saw no movement. They crossed directly in front of the group. Then a child whispered something. Immediately the elk crashed into the forest and out of view.

As the sound of breaking twigs died away, Everett said in a hushed tone, "Were those elk that I heard? Did I see some elk, Mommy?"

"Yes, Everett, you sure did," she replied, still a bit shaken by this bonus gift to the little ones.

Sunday of that first hunting weekend was October 31. Our kids had gladly forfeited the usual Halloween activities to come on the trip, but I brought a large pumpkin and some candies for their enjoyment. While dinner was being prepared, the children gathered around to witness surgery on the jack-o'-lantern. Then Everett Lee and Johnny Turner were costumed for trick-or-treating in paper-sack masks. This practice was unheard of in the wilderness, but we had noticed other children in a camp some distance from ours, so Jo Ann and Kathy took the two boys there to trick-or-treat.

The people were amazed, but they placed an apple and a candy bar in each of the boys' sacks. An hour later we observed flashlights coming toward our camp from the neighboring site. Three of their little people, with fresh paper-sack masks, were being escorted to trick-or-treat us. The candle-lighted pumpkin face grinned approvingly from a pickup canopy as we gave them goodies. None of us had expected this much Halloween fun in such an out-of-the-way place. The kids hadn't missed anything, after all, by joining in the family hunt.

Later the same evening, Lee Dimmick and I prepared a large bonfire for our worship service. The seven children and nine adults gathered around the fire for praise and songs under the stars.

"Let's sing 'Oh, How I Love Jesus,'" Everett Lee urged.

Steve accompanied this song and many others on his guitar. From time to time a family of coyotes supplied additional accompaniment. Diane and Steve sang several duets. Later than any of us realized, we joined in a final chorus of "I'm So Glad I'm Part of the Family of God." The Lord entered into this outdoor chapel and made it a genuine sanctuary. In the warm glow of the Spirit of God, we retired to tents and trailers.

Those days were full of the enjoyment we had all looked forward to for so long, but eventually a problem developed. We noticed Everett Lee holding his head at dinner one night. For three or four months he had been having moments of complaint about headaches. This seemed like more of the same, only worse. Mary Lee and I recognized that we would have to take him home immediately. Perhaps he just had a flu bug, but his shunt might be malfunctioning. It had been almost five years since the apparatus had plugged, and we were nearly convinced that he didn't need it any longer. However, we couldn't take any chances.

Within 30 minutes Mary Lee and our two girls were ready to leave with Everett. Fred and I remained behind to break camp and transport the equipment home. The state police knew our camp location and would inform us if Everett's condition worsened.

Everett Lee was alert, but clearly not well. Just as we were about to load him into the car for the five-hour drive to Portland, he stopped us. "Don't you think we should have prayer?" he asked.

"Yes, Everett, we should," I replied.

We had intended to do just that, but he was way ahead of us. And then he beat us to the punch again! Before Mary Lee or I could open our mouths, he led the six of us in prayer: "Our dear heavenly Father, thank you for letting me be here. And thank you for letting us have a good time. Please help us get home safely, and help me get well. In Jesus' name. Amen."

Standing around him in the door of the tent, with tears in our eyes, we all said, "Amen, Father. Amen."

CHAPTER EIGHTEEN

Thanksgiving Finale

*I*F A HIGHWAY were a living thing, how very many stories it would have to tell. Most cars and trucks speed along its surface in routine travel, but on most days, that highway could also observe errands of high interest. It could reveal emotions ranging from extreme happiness to grave fear.

As we sped toward Portland once again, these thoughts came to my mind. A week had passed since our return from the hunting trip. Everett Lee had improved, so the doctor had not found it necessary to hospitalize him. He had been able to return to school.

Yet things did not seem right. On several mornings Everett, who was no complainer, complained about headaches. Arriving home from school, he would sleep on the couch each evening for two or more hours. Such listlessness was not normal.

The doctor instructed us to watch closely and bring him in, should anything more develop. On this morning additional signals of excessive pressure were present. After four years of respite, we were making another of our well-worn "ambulance runs."

Many things seemed strangely like an instant replay. Yet, as Mary Lee held our limp son, I was impressed by how very much larger he was. Everett had indeed become a big boy. God had granted so much to us in nearly nine and a half years. Abundant colors of joys and blessings had filled in the dark splashes of pain and tensions on the canvas. God majestically painted Everett's life picture so the dark strokes only highlighted the beauty. Now, as before, we could simply turn over his life and needs to God.

The rising brickwork of Good Samaritan Hospital reminded me of 1 Samuel 7:12. Samuel set a large stone in a prominent location and named it Ebenezer. He attached this meaning to it: "Thus far the Lord has helped us." We could claim the same truth as we entered this monument of healing. God had shown himself to be an ever-present source of help. We knew he would not let us down now.

From our entry into the emergency room and on through the next eight days, the doctors were perplexed. In earlier experiences, all the readings and symptoms had been very clear. However, this time, some tests indicated one thing while some indicated another. Everett's condition fluctuated widely in the space of a few hours. He was scheduled for surgery three times, and then it was postponed twice. Because radical stresses would be involved, the doctors did not want to do a full shunt revision unless it was absolutely necessary. We were thankful that they did not overreact, that Everett would not be put through the pain and shock of surgery if it was not essential.

For parts of these days, Everett Lee was very chipper, carrying on a teasing warfare with the nurses and enjoying his roommate or visitors. But a short time later his eyes would reflect pain, and he would be disinterested in his surroundings. We did not understand what was causing the extreme changes in his moods and feelings.

Later we learned that the shunt had not been functioning properly for over a year. Unexplainably, Everett Lee had survived to experience many happy events with family and friends. During the entire hospitalization, he was much more ill than his physicians or parents knew.

When we had absorbed this information, we thought back on that borrowed year. Occurrences from the last several months suddenly fit into place. We attached the word "miracle" to the strength and health allowing him to experience so many joys. The testimony of his life in that time took on additional sparkle. And his words in the tent doorway were more piercing than before: "Dear heavenly Father, thank you for letting me be here."

Everett Lee's spirit of gratitude gleamed from the hospital bed. He showed great appreciation for the new pair of pajamas that replaced the ones he had worn to the hospital. Get-well cards were enjoyed again and again. He was thrilled by the cards special-delivered from his O.S.B. classmates. These messages were taped to the wall, and the greetings were read to visitors, with a running introduction of each card's author.

Good Samaritan Hospital no longer had the familiar pediatrics department. Everett was on the regular neurological floor in a typical adult two-bed ward. He was grateful that a kind man from Astoria, Oregon, occupied the other bed.

Bill Foster had arrived the same day as Everett Lee. This fine family man and community leader was enduring the intermittent early symptoms of a brain tumor. He showed special thoughtfulness in many ways to his young roommate.

One afternoon Mr. Foster asked, "Would you like an ice-cream sundae, Everett?"

"Yes!"

Bill sent his wife on a journey through the neighborhood in search of good ice-cream sundaes. She knew what to look for, because for many years Bill had run a fountain-drug store and had made the "best sundaes in three counties!"

Nearly an hour later Mrs. Foster returned with three good-sized, chocolate-drenched sundaes. I was glad to be included in this delicious treat. A few moments later we three happy consumers greeted the nurse as she entered the room. She surveyed the apologetic grins of the two men and the laughing boy. As she turned to leave, she told us: "Enjoy your sundaes, *boys!*"

The staff were all new to us, and we missed our friends of the old pediatrics ward. But Everett Lee was thankful for each of these wonderful people. He loved the young nurses who played his word games and the aides who sat on the bed to acquire information. Also, a roommate 40 years older who consulted him about television program selection was very special.

The extra efforts of people who stayed at his bedside drew expressions of thanks. On days when Mary Lee could not stay, Aunt Jo or Aunt Sharon, Kathy Dimmick, or Daddy was with him in the sometimes pleasant and sometimes painful hours. The homes of Mary Lee's sisters and my parents were constantly opened to our family. During Everett Lee's many illnesses, these relatives apparently gave little or no thought to the disruption of their lives or the invasion of their privacy. Together with us this boy was thankful for the kindnesses of loved ones.

One day when Kathy Dimmick was his attendant, Everett learned a new skill. Always before in the children's ward, he had been given liquid or chewable medications. Now some medications were not available in those forms. Kathy worked with him until he was successful in swallowing the necessary pills. Thereafter, Everett proudly displayed his new talent. He could hardly wait to show or tell: "Did you know I can swallow pills now?"

The medications temporarily relieved the pain of headaches and other symptoms of intense pressure in his head. Tests continued to be confusing. The doctors carefully watched for clarification. On Tuesday evening Dr. Raaf informed us, "We have scheduled the operating room for 9:00 A.M. Friday. It is now certain that the shunt is the culprit. We will do a complete revision." We were glad for a definite course of action at last.

Thanksgiving Day would precede the surgery. Since Everett appeared to be feeling quite well during part of each day, we considered taking him out of the hospital for a few hours to enjoy Thanksgiving dinner at Grandma's. However, we decided against moving him.

The day of national thanks was cloudy and cold. Twice Everett asked if it was snowing outside yet. Some persons in the room didn't know why that was important to him. Mary Lee and I did. He was still looking forward to keeping our appointment with a snowbank!

The other three kids and I spent an hour at the hospital before leaving for my folks' house. Mary Lee stayed with Everett. Turkey and all the trimmings were featured on both Grandma's table and the hospital menu. Throughout the day, we shifted from one locality to another.

A 17-year-old girl named Miriam was spending the holiday in the hospital, also. She had been in a room down the hall for three weeks, and she expected to be there several more. The two young people on this floor had met when she came into Everett's room to visit Bill Foster. She had known the Fosters for a long time. When she first guided her wheelchair into the room, we were warmed by her smile and friendship. This girl, a victim of a serious nerve disease, charmed us all by her happy disposition.

Miriam had constructed a very large greeting card which the nurses' aides affixed to the door of her room for Thanksgiving Day. As people entered she asked them to sign the card, naming the things for which they were thankful.

Before the holiday meal was served, Mary Lee accompanied Everett on a little walk. Stopping at Miriam's room, he was asked to write on the card. With no hesitation, he took the pen and printed the foremost object of his gratitude:

I'm thankful for the Lord

This expression from his heart was written in pain, with great care. He was suffering, yet the words were legible. The summary of his grateful spirit was thanksgiving for the giver of every good thing and every perfect gift. Unmistakably, Everett knew who had been so very good to him.

Later in the day our family united around his bed. Aunts and uncles and cousins stood sharing the unusual Thanksgiving with us. None of this assembly could have guessed the degree of seriousness of Everett's illness, for even in his present condition, he tried to add humor to the group. Once Everett held up the napkin from the meal tray. A colorful turkey was pictured on it. Everett said, "C.J., your daddy is one of these!"

"Turkey" meant foolish or stupid in current teen vernacular. With C.J.'s dad standing beside him, Everett repeated, "I think Roger is one of these!" Roger laughed the loudest at Everett's teasing.

As we began moving toward the door, we intended to encourage Everett Lee, but instead, he tried hard to entertain us. Jo Ann, Kathy, Fred, and I kissed him good-bye. It was obvious that he was not at all well. Mary Lee lingered in the hall, waving as we moved to the elevator. She would be spending the night with him. As she returned to his bedside, Everett quickly asked her to turn the light off. He whimpered slightly about a terrible headache.

In the darkened room she led him in reciting the verses from our life notebooks. He had more trouble than usual, but quoted verse after verse from the Word of God. Though his head was "swimming" and he complained of pain, these promises calmed and gave peace.

Of the surgery planned for the next morning, he said, "I'm not afraid, because I'm Everett. I'm strong and brave." Then he began the same prayer we had heard for years at bedtime: "Now I lay me down to sleep, I pray the Lord my soul to keep. If I should die before I wake, I pray the Lord my soul to take. God bless Mommy and Daddy, Fred, Jo Ann, and Kathy; C.J., and Mary Ellen, Steven, and Sharon Lee . . ." (and others of our extended family and friends). He concluded with:

"And dear God, please help Darlene Woodruff to

get over her sore back and help Bill Foster get better, and help me get well. In Jesus' name. Amen."

Those next few hours were filled with great pain. Everett Lee experienced hallucinations of "spinning like a top," and we saw other glimpses of feelings experienced by an overpressured brain. The medications seemed to be of no help, but finally Everett went to sleep. In a chair next to his bed, Mary Lee too fell asleep, with the surgery only five hours away.

Something prompted me to be at the hospital by 7:00 A.M. I was met in the hall by Sharon Beeson, who, like her sister Shirley Harpool, had become like our own daughter. An inner prompting had told her the 7:00 A.M. hour as well. We could see Mary Lee and Everett asleep in the room still dimmed by drawn venetian blinds. To avoid disturbing them, we visited in the hall.

Moments later Dr. Raaf, with two other doctors and Ruby Waterston, came down the hall for a routine check on the patient scheduled for surgery in less than two hours. They greeted us and then stepped into the room. Mary Lee awoke as the lights were turned on. The group first spoke to her. Then moving to the bed the doctors made the startling discovery. Everett Lee was gone!

We were quickly ushered out. The hospital emergency code was sounded. Amid the flurry of running feet and rolling wheels, Mary Lee, Sharon, and I stood weeping and praying. We comforted each other by words and by touch. Minutes later we were seated in a tiny room. Dr. Raaf and Ruby had tears running down their cheeks, too. Overcome with shock, they shared love and sorrow with us. They had accepted Everett Lee into their hearts, and all of us had accepted Dr. Raaf and Ruby into ours.

It was some time before the door opened and the five of us stepped out of that little office. Much silent prayer had ascended from the grieved and burdened people in that room. God was present in a very real way. He had not forsaken us.

"God just didn't want him to endure another of those surgeries."

"The gift of his life was very good. Now Everett Lee's death must be accepted as a good gift from a kind and loving heavenly Father."

Everett had prayed, "If I should die before I wake, I pray the Lord my soul to take." We knew that God had taken our son's spirit to his eternal heavenly home. Yet the trip down the elevator and through the halls to the car was the most painful I have ever experienced. Mary Lee and I have never known greater loneliness than when leaving the hospital without our baby for the last time.

We prayed, "Father, thank you for all the good gifts you have given to Everett Lee and to us. Thank you for answering our prayers for him to be made completely whole. Please give us the comfort we need right now. Dear Father, please minister to us as we tell our kids of Everett's death. . . . And, Father, would you throw him into a snowbank for me, please?"

CHAPTER NINETEEN

Celebrating Victory

GOD DID MINISTER to us in the next hours and days in a wonderful way. Through tear-filled eyes we saw the words in Psalm 116:15: "Precious in the sight of the Lord is the death of His godly ones."

After a long 15-minute drive, Mary Lee and I arrived at my parents' house. Fred, Jo Ann, and Kathy were still asleep. I thought their hearts and ours would break when they awoke to the news. The love between them and their little brother had been mountain-size. The years of expressed and unexpressed joy in sharing his life was poured out like a burst dam.

Yet, in the midst of this grief, the death, burial, and resurrection of Jesus Christ made a great difference. The gospel was showing itself powerful. Faith in the risen Christ had filled our home, and each of us knew it had filled Everett Lee. We wept in each other's arms while praising God for the eyes and feet that now had been made perfect. The tears were for painful absence, but not for permanent loss. The boy whom we had been privileged to have in our home had *run* to *see* Jesus in Hallelujah Square. One day we would meet at Jesus' feet.

After comforting one another, we drove to the beach for the weekend, for we needed time alone. I felt that brief retreat in the presence of God at the cabin by the sea would bring peace.

At first everyone was quiet as we drove. Then broken voices shared "the hope that is within us."

Fred said, "Everett Lee is better off than any of us now."

Commenting on the extreme suffering he had experienced in the hours before dawn, Mary Lee added, "We wouldn't wish him back from the glory of heaven, even if we could."

We began to shape plans for the funeral. It would be in the church building. The songs Everett had loved so dearly would be sung. Glen Lyda from Camp Wi-Ne-Ma was the entire family's choice to bring the message. It would be a praise service, witnessing to a celebration of victory.

As we drove, we prayed, "Father, please guide us in planning and preparing for Everett Lee's funeral. Make it according to your will. We want it to speak loudly of the victory won by Jesus for us over death. May you receive glory and honor in his death, as you did by his life."

That weekend we received visits from three families. Larry and Judy Parmley, Glen and Elaine Lyda, and Lee and Kathy Dimmick, with their daughters Cindy and Wendy, brought love and understanding. God sent these "like family" friends into our private time of sorrow.

During the retreat days, a vacancy was prominent in our little assembly, but we reminded ourselves that the Payton family still numbered six. The empty place in our family circle belonged to the boy who had gone on ahead to our heavenly home.

In those hours we experienced the difference that eternal hope makes. "But we do not want you to be uninformed, brethren, about those who are asleep, that you may not grieve, as do the rest who have no hope. For if we believe that Jesus died and rose again, even so God will bring with Him those who have fallen asleep in Jesus" (1 Thess. 4:13-14).

With the approach of the funeral, we prayed that the service and our lives would reflect that difference. Once again we invited the Lord into our weakness to show himself strong.

Half an hour before the appointed time on Tuesday morning, the church auditorium was filled. Chairs were placed in the aisles and in the foyer. Latecomers were seated in the classrooms down the hall.

Our church family was well represented from the four congregations we had pastored. Relatives filled the seats reserved for them and overflowed into one of the classrooms. There were many students from neighboring schools and the church youth groups.

The most striking sight was the human chain of unsighted children who came from the Oregon School for the Blind. Sorrow at the loss of this classmate was evident in their faces as teachers and administrators led them to reserved seats. They contributed in a major way to the service's being a proper tribute.

Carl Hemminger said, "This is the largest funeral I have ever seen in my 62 years." Later he also commented about our family's pause at the casket before being seated: "I thought my heart would explode within me. His mother tucked Everett Lee in for the last time, with a half-smile on her face. She knew full well that he was safely tucked into the arms of Jesus." The white casket was closed over the form of our son holding the cherished large-print New Testament.

God did grant Mary Lee and our three youngsters a special peace and strength. Then he allowed me the ability to lead in the first choruses sung by the congregation. The Spirit of God led us all to see the difference that Jesus Christ makes in the face of death.

The service was special. Several hundred persons sang the choruses and hymns. Steve and Diane Turner, accompanied on guitar and organ, sang beautiful duets. The Scripture verses and Glen's message focused on victory through Jesus over sin, Satan, and the grave. Everett Lee's happy testimony of life and faith were noted, with the glory given to God for this miracle life.

As our family followed the casket up the aisle, the congregation sang, "Let's Just Praise the Lord." Those 45 minutes had indeed been a tribute to a boy and his heavenly Father. The chorus of praise was sung repeatedly as all left the building. Few left untouched by a miracle of peace and strength.

Warm embraces and words of sympathy filled the next few minutes. Then we began the 25-mile drive to Amity, a small community located between Salem and McMinnville. My mother's family were early settlers in that area. The picturesque old cemetery on the edge of town contains the remains of her forebears. One of the earliest buried here was a veteran of the War of 1812.

Except for eight years when I lived in California, I had been drawn to this cemetery and the adjacent park each Memorial Day. Knowledge of my heritage and roots came to me as I helped my grandparents and parents groom and decorate the graves. Every Memorial Day was a pleasant time for reunion and picnicking while returning to the soil from which we sprang. Every year I take my children to the earliest grave titled simply "Indian Jim," dating from 1840. My children place flowers on the grave just as I did as a child. Now, 20 yards from that most ancient headstone, a freshly dug grave awaited us.

We had not expected many to make the trip to the graveside, but scores of cars respectfully trailed us. The serene, rolling farmland imparted a benediction on the procession. When we arrived at the west edge of the tiny town, the immense trees and large old monuments came into view. The discarded body of clay so identified with our son was lovingly brought to this place. We knew that Everett was not here, but our sentiment for this spot was much deepened because it now held his remains.

Glen Lyda read these verses of scripture: "[We know] that He who raised the Lord Jesus will raise us also with Jesus and will present us with you. . . . Therefore we do not lose heart, but though our outer man is decaying, yet our inner man is being renewed day by day. For momentary, light affliction is producing for us an eternal weight of glory far beyond all comparison, while we look not at the things which are seen, but at the things which are not seen; for the things which are seen are temporal, but the things which are not seen are eternal" (2 Cor. 4:14-18).

After the committal prayer of thanksgiving and praise to God for his eternal promises and for Everett Lee's life, all of us turned from the mound of flowers to one another. God had answered our prayers for this day in a very special way.

We left very grateful. Our family still numbered six! Our good heavenly Father had united us in his eternal family. Christians never see their loved ones for the last time. Everett Lee and we are united by everlasting love.

Time is . . .
Too slow for those who wait,
Too swift for those who fear,
Too long for those who grieve,
Too short for those who rejoice;
But for those who love,
Time is not.

—Henry Van Dyke

CHAPTER TWENTY

A Life of Song

Two MONTHS after Everett Lee's death, one boy put into words what many people were feeling. Oscar Ramone had been Everett's close friend at the Oregon School for the Blind. In late January Mrs. Summers took a new student to what had been Everett's desk. The newcomer had just sat down when Oscar, in a no-nonsense tone, ordered, "Get up! That is Everett Lee's place."

Most certainly no one could fill Everett's place for any of us. His life had radiated in song. The words and melody might have been sad, but instead he produced glad ones. By God's grace, Mary Lee and I had helped to direct this beautiful "broken doll." We certainly didn't have all the answers. We were learners, and not always good students at that. But we found God faithful and available to cheer and to guide us.

Everett Lee's life verse was a constant reminder. God firmly commits himself in Joshua 1:9: "Have I not commanded you? Be strong and courageous! Do not tremble or be dismayed, for the Lord your God is with you wherever you go."

Another of Everett's memory verses that helped point our family toward victory is John 16:33. Jesus says, "These things I have spoken to you, that in Me you may have peace. In the world you have tribulation, but take courage; I have overcome the world."

Of necessity we spent many sleepless nights during our son's illnesses. But other nights and days were filled with tension under an unnecessary burden of anxiety. We had given Everett's needs to the Lord, but we were trying to "help God out," carrying the load ourselves. God expects us to expend ourselves in serving loved ones, but the prescription of faith will always produce peace. Our tribulation may be strenuous and exhausting, but the Lord wants us to meet it with a cheerful, victorious spirit. Only when we look to Jesus Christ and trust him in every situation can victory result.

This truth is expressed very well in another of Bill and Gloria Gaither's songs. It was one of Everett Lee's favorites.

Because He Lives

God sent His Son, They called Him Jesus,
He came to love . . . heal and forgive;
He lived and died to buy my pardon,
An empty grave is there
to prove my Savior Lives.

How sweet to hold our new born baby,
And feel the pride and joy He gives;
But greater still the calm assurance,
This child can face uncertain days
    because He Lives.

And then one day I'll cross the river,
I'll fight life's final war with pain;
And then as death gives way to victory,
I'll see the lights of glory
    and I'll know He Reigns.

Chorus:
Because He Lives I can face tomorrow,
Because He Lives all fear is gone;
Because I know He holds the future,
And life is worth the living,
Just because He Lives.

None of us knows how much pain Everett Lee felt inside his hydrocephalic head. On some days it must have been incredible. We can only guess how that arm and leg ached while balking at every movement. He also hurt when he fell over unseen objects while trying to keep up with other kids. But through it all, he found God trustworthy. In the death of Jesus on a cruel cross, God had reached out purchasing salvation for Everett. Then the Spirit of God who raised that same Jesus to life gave victorious life to this boy. The truth, "God is so good to me," was the source of his song of happiness.

The junior choir director said, "Oh, how I'll miss Everett's voice in the choir!"

Our Kathy responded, "He's up in heaven singing in his loud, magnificent voice. He's running like the other boys and seeing perfectly God's glorious heaven. Our loss is heaven's gain."

God trusted our family with a very special life. Mom and Dad, sisters and brother had all gone through pain with Everett. Burdens and pressures had been plentiful. But through them all, each of us had found God to be faithful and worthy of our trust. The extra investments of time and energy had paid big dividends. This special package from heaven had clearly illustrated lessons of love and faith and service. Truly Everett Lee was a perfect gift to our home.

He was a good gift to many others, also. Through him, scores of people received blessings from God. Merle and Dexter Maust summarized the mark his life had made. "He was like a gigantic patch of sunshine," Merle said. Dexter told friends, "Everett Lee's life touched more people for the Lord than many pastors ever do."

What is the real value of a life, anyway? One of the measures would have to be the amount of blessing brought to others. God has shown us that special lives multiply special blessings. We are forever grateful.

"Father, thank you for giving Everett Lee to us. And thank you that he lives because Jesus lives."

A final prayer from our house to yours: "Now may our God and Father Himself and Jesus our Lord direct our way to you; and may the Lord cause you to increase and abound in love for one another, and for all men, just as we also do for you; so that He may establish your hearts unblamable in holiness before our God and Father at the coming of our Lord Jesus with all His saints (1 Thess. 3:11-13).